Neurobehavioral Consequences of Closed Head Injury

Neurobehavioral Consequences of Closed Head Injury

HARVEY S. LEVIN, PH.D.
Division of Neurosurgery
The University of Texas Medical Branch
Galveston, Texas

ARTHUR L. BENTON, PH.D.
Departments of Neurology and Psychology
University of Iowa
Iowa City, Iowa

ROBERT G. GROSSMAN, M.D.
Department of Neurosurgery
Baylor College of Medicine
Houston, Texas

New York   Oxford
OXFORD UNIVERSITY PRESS
1982

Library of Congress Cataloging in Publication Data

Levin, Harvey S.
  Neurobehavioral consequences of closed head injury.

  Bibliography: p.
  Includes index.
    1. Brain — Wounds and injuries — Complications and
sequelae.   2. Cognition disorders.   3. Personality,
Disorders of.   I. Benton, Arthur Lester, 1909–
II. Grossman, Robert G.   III. Title.   IV. Title: Closed
head injury. [DNLM: 1. Brain injuries, Acute–Psychol-
ogy. WL 354 L665n]
RD594.L46   617'.48107   81-16777
ISBN 0-19-503008-7   AACR2

Printing (last digit):   9 8 7 6 5

Printed in the United States of America

To the Memory of
W. Ritchie Russell

Preface

Our purpose in writing this monograph has been to present a critical summary of current knowledge about the behavioral consequences of traumatic head injury, particularly closed head injury. It is based primarily on research findings rather than on impressions emerging from clinical experience. This bias reflects our conviction that only systematic controlled study that takes account of the numerous factors that determine the nature of the behavioral and social outcome of head injury can provide the basic knowledge necessary for its rational management and effective rehabilitation.

The personal, social, and economic consequences of head injuries, particularly those resulting from automobile accidents, assaults, and athletic mishaps, can scarcely be overestimated. Thanks to the remarkable life-saving capabilities of modern neurosurgical management of acute severe head injuries, the number of patients surviving such injuries mounts steadily. However, the great majority of these patients do not survive unscathed. Instead, they are left with residual cerebral damage that may impair intellectual functioning and emotional stability, and these impairments seriously affect their personal and economic adjustment. Hence, in recent years, the focus of interest has shifted, to a considerable degree, from the fact of survival to the question of the *quality* of survival of the posttraumatic patient.

Cognitive defects and emotional disturbances, as well as global "personality changes" that sometimes defy precise description, have always been recognized as prominent sequelae of the acute phase of traumatic head injury. At the same time, there is now general agreement that a posttraumatic patient's cognitive and emotional status is at least as powerful a determinant of his personal and social competence as his physical status. As a result, such questions as the characteristic features of the course of recovery from brain damage, the factors that influence the rate and extent of recovery, the specific cognitive functions that are most seriously impaired, the prognostic significance of anatomic, physiologic, and behavioral observations during the early stages of recovery, the relationship of cognitive and emotional disturbance to life adjustment, and the development of effective programs of rehabilitation have become issues of paramount importance in the field. Each of them is currently the subject of active investigative interest.

The initial impetus for writing this book was our own felt need, as workers in the field, for an integrated summary of what is known, what is not known, and what should be ascertained. We have learned much from the effort. On the one hand, we have come to appreciate that, despite the important substantive and methodological advances that have been achieved during the past decade, current knowledge is still of rather limited clinical value when applied to the individual patient. On the other hand, some specific directions future research should take have been identified. Thus, the product of our labors has performed a useful service to us. We hope that it will perform the same useful service to the interested reader.

We are most grateful to Dr. Howard M. Eisenberg and Dr. Ellen M. Levin for their careful reading of the manuscript and their many helpful suggestions. We are also indebted to Sarah A. De Los Santos and Julie Gips for their patience and skill in typing the manuscript and to Mr. David A. Hulkonen, of the Moody Medical Library, for providing much valuable reference material.

The authors' own research, which is cited in various places in the book, was supported by Program Project Grant DHEW 5P01 NS-07377, Comprehensive Trauma Center Contract NO1 NS 9-2314 and Research Grant NS-00616 from the National Institute of Neurological and Communicative Disorders and Stroke.

We dedicate this book to the memory of Dr. W. Ritchie Russell, whose groundbreaking studies of closed head injury and the effects of penetrating brain wounds provided an indispensable basis for the subsequent advancement of knowledge and understanding in this field.

Galveston   H.S.L.
Iowa City   A.L.B.
Houston   R.G.G.
April 1981

Contents

Neurobehavioral Consequences of Closed Head Injury

1. Pathophysiologic mechanisms

Historical review of head injury

This section covers only a few highlights in the development of knowledge of the mechanisms and behavioral consequences of head trauma. The interested reader will find detailed accounts of the historical evolution of facts and theories in the field in the writings of Strauss and Savitsky (1934), Mettler (1945), Courville (1953), Benton and Joynt (1960), and Gurdjian (1973).

Head injuries must have been very common in the life of primitive people, given the harsh and dangerous conditions of their existence, and they must have been quite familiar with some of the consequences of these injuries. There is clear evidence in the oldest known medical document, the Edwin Smith Surgical Papyrus (itself a copy of an older manuscript written about 3000 B.C.), that the ancient Egyptians were aware that injuries to the skull and brain caused diverse disturbances of function (Breasted, 1930). For example, cases of paraplegia and speechlessness following left temporal depressed skull fracture are described in the Papyrus.

Most ancient Greek physicians and philosophers regarded the brain as the central organ for perception and thought, a conclusion almost certainly based on observations of patients who had sustained head injuries. Alcmaeon of Croton (*ca.* 500 B.C.), for example, held that "the brain furnished the sensations of hearing, sight, and smelling, from which memory and judgment are born, and from these sensations, once established, wisdom is also born" (Castiglioni, 1958).

Alcmaeon conceived of the nerves as being canals that connected the sense organs with the brain and hence served the function of conveying information to it.

The physicians of the Hippocratic school (*ca.* 400 B.C.) made the important observation that "an incised wound in one temple produces a spasm in the opposite side of the body" (Chadwick and Mann, 1950). They were also quite aware that disturbances in speech and language were frequent sequelae of brain damage. That head trauma could cause highly specific disabilities was demonstrated by Valerius Maximus (*ca.* A.D. 30) in his description of alexia in a learned man who was struck in the head by a stone and "lost his memory of letters, to which he had been particularly devoted, but retained his memory of everything else." Later Galen (130–200) noted that a specific "loss of memory for words" may follow head injury (Major, 1954).

An anatomic basis for the Hippocratic rule that a blow on one side of the head causes motor impairment on the opposite side of the body was offered by Aretaeus of Cappadocia. The chapter on paralysis in his treatise on chronic diseases includes the following passage:

> If, therefore, the commencement of the affection be below the head, such as the membrane of the spinal marrow, the parts which are homonymous and connected with it are paralyzed, the right on the right side, and the left on the left side. But if the head be primarily affected on the right side, the left side of the body will be paralyzed; and the right, if on the left side. The cause of this is the interchange in the origin of the nerves, for they do not pass along on the same side, the right on the right side, until their terminations; but each of them passes over to the other side from that of its origin, decussating each other in the form of the letter X (Adams, 1856).

This remarkable early formulation of the rule of contralateral innervation was generally ignored by later generations of physicians. Perhaps it was not even known to most of them. Only in the 18th century was its validity established beyond doubt by the experimental demonstration by Pourfour du Petit (1710) of the crossing of the pyramidal tracts and by the clinicopathologic correlations of Morgagni (1769).

Surgical intervention to alleviate the consequences of traumatic head injury dates back to prehistoric times and in fact trepanation of the skull is "the most ancient operation of which we have objective evidence" (Castiglioni, 1958). The reasons for this extraordinarily widespread practice—ancient trepanned skulls have been found on every continent—remain conjectural. It appears that headache, depressed skull fracture and demonic possession were the most frequent indications. The Hippocratic writings include descriptions of head injuries and directions for trepanation. Greek and Roman surgeons trepanned for head wounds, developed instruments for removing bone fragments after trepanation, and repaired scalp lacerations. Further technical advances were reflected in the practice of medieval surgeons, such as Roger of Salerno (12th century), whose treatise included considerations of the differential diagnosis of head and brain wounds and the indications for trepanation. "For depressed fractures, it is recommended to make a number of holes with the trephine and then slowly raise the fractured bone without damaging the meninges" (Castiglioni, 1958). This general plan of management was continued until the development of antiseptic and aseptic surgery.

Renaissance surgeons, such as Ambroise Paré (1510–1540), Nicolò Massa (d. 1569), and Francisco Arceo (1493–1573), continued this development. Arceo (1598), for example, described his management of a construction worker who was hit on the head by a falling stone. Parts of the skull were depressed into the brain and for some days after the accident the patient was speechless. Arceo deflected the bone fragments into place and, in doing this, observed that the meninges were inflamed. Three days later, the patient began to speak (at first "imperfecklie and as men of troubled minde are wonte to do"), but eventually he recovered completely. Gurdjian (1973) records that Hieronymous Brunschwig (1450–1533) and John De Vigo (1450–1525) were the first to report cases of gunshot wounds to the brain.

Contrecoup fractures following head injury were among the different types of fractures mentioned in the Hippocratic writings. Later authors, such as Ambroise Paré, described contrecoup injuries of the meninges and brain substance. The nature of the physical mechanisms producing contrecoup lesions became a topic of intense interest in the 18th century, particularly in France, and numerous theories were advanced. There is still debate among neurosurgeons about different aspects of the problem. Other developments in the 18th century included studies of intracranial pressure and swelling of the brain. Surgical evacuation of epidural hematomas was practiced, but intradural hematomas were thought to be inoperable. John Abernethy (1764–1831) concluded that extravasation between the dura and the skull was the only indication for use of the trephine. Conservative therapy of head injury included blood letting and the administration of purgatives.

The management of head injury did not change appreciably during the 19th century, although knowledge of lesions in various structures of the brain was enhanced by pathologic studies. Gurdjian (1973) notes that mortality from penetrating wounds of the brain, which approached 90% in antiquity, remained very high during the Napoleonic and Crimean wars. Gurdjian traces contemporary neurosurgical management of head injury to the teachings of Joseph Lister (1827–1912) on antiseptic surgery.

Although posttraumatic concussion or comotio cerebri, i.e., gross derangement of cerebral function without obvious structural damage to the brain, was familiar to laymen and physicians alike, its symptoms were first described in a systematic fashion by Berengario da Carpi in the 16th century. Both he and Paré ascribed concussion to intracranial bleeding, an opinion that found support centuries later in the findings by Duret (1878) of microscopic hemorrhages in the brains of patients who had died after severe cerebral concussion. J.L. Petit, in the 18th century, distinguished between concussion, contusion, and compression of the brain resulting from head injury. Concussion, he felt, was due to the transmission of the vibrations of the skull to the substance of the brain and he made the observation that the effect was more severe if the skull had not been fractured.

The paradox of the occurrence of severe functional disturbances within the setting of negative, or at most minimal, anatomic findings preoccupied the attention of 19th-century physicians who were seeing an increasing number of traumatic cases of different types with the rapid industrialization of society and the growth of railway transportation. Some advanced a physiologic explanation of the phenomenon, a favored concept being that of "molecular disarrangement." Gamma (1835) anticipated modern histologic studies when he postulated that "fibers as delicate as those of which the organ of mind is composed are liable to break as a result of violence to the head."

Experimental studies of blunt injury to the central nervous system were published in the 19th century and during the early part of the 20th century. Strich (1956) cites the work of Schmaus (1890–1899), who demonstrated that secondary degeneration of nerve fibers occurs above and below the level of injury. Schmaus inferred that nerve fibers die as a result of mechanical damage. This early contribution was confirmed and extended by Strich's classic studies of injury to the cerebral white matter.

Case studies of recovery after closed head injury, published by English physicians and surgeons during the latter half of the 19th century, have been recently reviewed by Levin, Peters, and Hulkonen (1982). These reports, which provided detailed descriptions of anterograde amnesia, were cited by Ribot (1882) in his theoretical formulations of amnesia and the organization of normal memory. Clinical studies of head injury published after the turn of the century extended the earlier findings in characterizing neuropsychiatric sequelae. In their discussions, these authors began to distinguish between preexisting behavioral tendencies and the effects of brain injury.

Implications of pathophysiologic mechanisms for neuropsychology

Investigators have traditionally studied the relationship between cerebral local-ization of lesion and neuropsychological deficit in patients with occlusion of the cerebral blood vessels. These patients offer the opportunity to evaluate the effects of a circumscribed area of brain damage over a long period of time. Although computed tomographic (CT) scanning in patients with nontrivial head injury frequently visualizes a focal brain contusion or intracranial hema-toma confined to a single hemisphere, as a general rule this lesion is superim-posed on a diffuse cerebral injury of varying severity. An emerging theme of recent neuropathologic studies is that the primary mechanism of closed head injury is mechanical shearing/stretching of nerve fibers immediately on impact (cf. Adams, Mitchell, Graham, and Doyle, 1977). As will be seen, efforts to relate the intrahemispheric site of mass lesion in head-injured patients to the pattern of neuropsychological deficit have been complicated by widespread micro-scopic injury to nerve fibers that is not fully disclosed by CT imaging. Moreover, diffuse white matter injury may produce asymmetric damage to the cerebral hemispheres and fiber tracts (Adams et al., 1977) and produce a lateralized neu-ropsychological deficit in apparent contradiction to CT findings that are com-patible with diffuse injury or a mass lesion situated in the opposite hemisphere.

In contrast to visualization of focal brain lesions by CT and surgical findings, the severity of diffuse cerebral injury after closed head trauma must be assessed indirectly by measuring the impairment of neurologic function. Progress in using physiologic measures (e.g., cerebral blood flow, evoked potentials) to eval-uate the severity of hemispheric injury and the integrity of the brain stem may also elucidate the mechanisms of injury and recovery (Greenberg et al., 1977; Obrist et al., 1979).

The classification of closed head injury severity, which is essential for neu-robehavioral studies of outcome, has been substantially revised as a result of recent clinical and pathologic investigations, which are reviewed in this chapter. These studies have provided support for a spectrum of closed head injury in which injuries differ quantitatively (e.g., degree of shearing of nerve fibers). Bakay and Glasauer (1980) note that concussion has been traditionally charac-terized as a "brief loss of consciousness followed by prompt recovery and with-out any localizing neurologic signs." The authors point out that it was generally thought in the past that "no visible anatomic changes occur in the concussed brain, the whole syndrome being functional in nature.". As will be seen, this view of minor head injury has been called into question by pathologic evidence of microscopic lesions after mild head injury and neuropsychologic findings indicating that concussed patients exhibit a transient reduction in information-processing efficiency concomitant with characteristic behavioral symptoms that appear to be cumulative, i.e., sequelae are more severe after a second minor head injury (Gronwall and Wrightson, 1975; Oppenheimer, 1968).

Notwithstanding the evidence for a spectrum of closed head injury severity, the heterogeneity of injury must be appreciated in neuropsychological studies. A comparable level of impaired consciousness may be observed in patients who differ considerably in brain pathology (e.g., brain herniation secondary to an expanding epidural hematoma as contrasted to severe diffuse injury to the cerebral white matter). Although we recognize the complex problem of classifying the severity of closed head injury, in this chapter we review recent advances in the quantitative assessment of coma and in the neuroradiologic imaging of brain pathology that have facilitated neuropsychological research.

Mechanisms of impact

The two major types of head injury are missile injury (e.g., gunshot wounds) and nonmissile or closed head injury. Blunt trauma to the head results either from the impact of a moving object upon a stationary or slower moving head (acceleration) or when the head and body are decelerated by a stationary or slower moving object (Gurdjian, 1971). Linear and rotational acceleration typically coexist or follow one another in closed head injury. Blunt trauma to the head may injure the scalp, deform the skull with or without fracture, and shift the intracranial contents. Intracranial pressure appears to increase briefly on impact. Although blunt trauma associated with acceleration/deceleration forces to the head is the primary mechanism of impact in closed head injury, bone fragments can penetrate the brain tissue in cases of depressed skull fracture.

Penetrating missile injury, typically produced by gunshot or fragments from exploding shells, causes laceration of the scalp, perforation or fracture of the skull, and laceration of brain tissue in the path of the foreign body. A shower of bone fragments often penetrates the brain at the point of impact, the depth of dural penetration and loss of brain tissue representing indices of injury severity (Russell, 1947). Computed tomographic scanning provides visualization of the path of the missile as shown in Figure 1-1. Blood is also frequently seen in the basal cisterns, the interhemispheric fissure, and the ventricles.

Loss of consciousness

Impairment of consciousness is widely viewed as a characteristic feature of acute closed head injury, although prolonged loss of consciousness is relatively

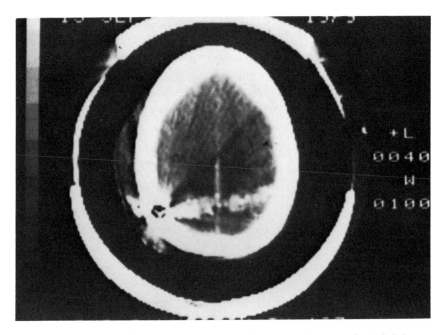

Fig. 1-1. Computerized tomographic scan visualizing gunshot wounds with left posterior parietal entry site. The path of the bullet is represented by a linear area of increased radiodensity; the bullet traversed the right posterior parietal area and then ricocheted to lodge in the right temporal lobe. There are isolated areas of bone loss in the left posterior frontal and parietal bone, related to the entry wounds. The CT scan was performed on the day of injury.

uncommon in consecutive head injury admissions to major trauma hospitals (Clifton, Grossman, Makela, Miner, Handel, and Sadhu, 1980). Coma, i.e., a state in which there is no eye opening, an inability to obey commands, and no utterance of recognizable words (Teasdale and Jennett, 1974), was found by Clifton and his colleagues to persist until the time of hospital admission in less than one-third of consecutive head-injured patients. The proportion of head-injured patients rendered comatose is even smaller if cases of minor closed head injuries discharged after treatment in the emergency room are included. Plum and Posner (1980) qualitatively distinguished clouding of consciousness, delirium, obtundation, and stupor from coma primarily on the basis that these altered states of consciousness are compatible with some preservation of psychologic responsiveness to the environment even if the patient must be aroused by vigorous and repeated stimuli. Although neuropsychological studies of closed head injury have often been focused on severe injuries followed by coma, there is increasing interest in the sequelae of head injuries that result in impairment, but not complete loss of consciousness (cf. Gronwall and Sampson, 1974).

Disruption of the reticular activating system of the rostral brain stem has been implicated in the onset of coma, although widespread injury to the cerebrum is usually concomitant (Plum and Posner, 1980). Rotation of the cerebrum around its junction with the midbrain, with consequent stretching of the reticular structures forming this junction, is presumed to be the primary cause of immediate loss of consciousness following head trauma (Martin, 1974). Paralysis of brain stem functioning at the onset of coma was confirmed in experimental studies of acceleration injury in animals (Denny-Brown and Russell, 1941). The authors observed that impact immediately disrupted respiratory and vasomotor responses (e.g., rise in blood pressure, peripheral vasoconstriction) and transient abolition of the corneal reflex and the pinna reflex (twitching or the ear when the anterior portion of the meatus is touched). From these observations, Denny-Brown and Russell defined concussion as the occurrence of "an immediate traumatic paralysis of reflex functioning, which occurs in the absence of lesions in the nervous system."

More recently, Ommaya and Gennarelli (1974) attributed traumatic unconsciousness to shear strain reaching the mesencephalic brain stem and causing a "disconnection of the alerting system of the brain." According to their postulation of a centripetal sequence of disruptive effects caused by blunt head injury, it follows that primary damage to the brain stem would not occur in isolation, but rather would always be a component of diffuse damage to the brain.

The assertion that primary brain stem damage does not occur in isolation from more widespread cerebral injury has been debated. Support for the Ommaya and Gennarelli view was provided by neuropathological studies completed in Glasgow (Adams et al., 1977; Mitchell and Adams, 1973) and in London (Crompton, 1971a). Macroscopic and histologic findings were reviewed in the brains of patients who were rendered unconscious immediately on impact and sustained diffuse cerebral damage, but with no indication of secondary brain stem injury, i.e., no evidence of raised intracranial pressure, herniation, or distortion of the brain. Primary impact damage to the brain stem in such cases was inferred from the finding of degenerative changes in the midbrain and pons. Patients who survived for several weeks or months had evidence of degeneration in the ascending or descending tracts of the brain stem. This finding was consistently accompanied by diffuse injury to the white matter of the cerebral hemispheres. Mitchell and Adams (1973) concluded that "the principal reason for the difficulty in defining primary localized brain stem damage due to blunt head injury is that it does not exist as a pathological entity."

Whereas unconsciousness produced immediately on impact in patients sustaining primary brain stem injury appears to result in concomitant diffuse injury to the cerebral white matter, traumatic hyperextension of the head may cause relatively specific contusional tears and hemorrhages in the rostral pyramids and adjacent structures at the junction of the medulla oblongata and pons (Lindenberg and Freytag, 1970). Although the authors reported that all cases had tears and hemorrhages at the pontomedullary junction and additional hemorrhages extended rostrally toward the tegmentum of the pons, the cerebrum was free of visible lesions in more than one-half the cases. Lindenberg and Freytag postulated that backward motion of the head mechanically induced tearing and stretching of fiber tracts at the time of impact. Midbrain injury, secondary to transtentorial herniation, can result in delayed impairment of consciousness.

Supratentorial mass lesions that encroach upon diencephalic structures also depress the level of consciousness. Although unilateral hemispheric lesions may produce an acute decrement in alertness depending upon their size and remote effects, Plum and Posner (1980) assert that coma requires "bilateral and extensive damage or dysfunction of the cerebral hemispheres or diencephalon." Other authors have implicated the role of diffuse brain injury in producing coma after nonmissile head trauma.

Animal models of blunt head injury have shown that traumatic unconsciousness results from impact to a free-moving head, which presumably causes rotational acceleration. Denny-Brown and Russell (1941) found that unconsciousness was produced immediately after impact when the skull was subjected to a sudden change in velocity, i.e., "acceleration concussion." The authors reported that a much greater force was necessary to produce unconsciousness when an animal's head was in a fixed position as compared to when it was free to move. Employing a device in which acceleration was imparted to the head of a rhesus monkey through a helmet, Ommaya and Gennarelli (1974) tested the rotational and linear components separately using identical levels of force. The authors reported that head shaking, which was primarily rotational, consistently resulted in intracranial hematomas and loss of consciousness, whereas linear acceleration (i.e., movement in a straight line) produced circumscribed brain lesions, but no coma.

Pathology of closed head injury

The discussion of the pathology of closed head injury is organized into sections on focal brain lesions and diffuse cerebral injury. Secondary effects of closed head injury listed in Table 1-1 are differentiated from primary mechanisms of injury in the following sections, although clinical studies and neuropathological

Table 1-1. Primary and secondary brain injury after closed head trauma

Primary (immediate on impact) brain injury
A. Macroscopic lesions
  1. Contusions underlying the site of impact (coup)
  2. Contrecoup contusion frequently in the undersurfaces of the frontal lobes and the tips of the temporal lobes
  3. Laceration of the brain from depressed skull fracture
B. Microscopic lesions
  1. Widespread shearing/stretching of nerve fibers

Secondary mechanisms of brain injury
A. Intracranial hemorrhage
B. Edema in white matter adjacent to focal mass lesions
C. Diffuse brain swelling—hyperemia
D. Ischemic brain damage
E. Raised intracranial pressure
F. Brain shift and herniation

Secondary insult from extracerebral events
A. Effects of multiple/systemic injury
  1. Hypoxia
  2. Fat embolism

Delayed effects
A. Degeneration of white matter
B. Disturbed flow of cerebrospinal fluid—hydrocephalus

evidence indicate that these combine and interact to result in marked heterogeneity of injury.

Mechanisms of diffuse injury

There is mounting evidence that diffuse cerebral injury produced at the moment of impact is the primary mechanism of brain damage in closed head injury patients (Adams et al., 1977; Strich, 1956, 1970). Moreover, the severity of diffuse brain injury is a more important determinant of the quality of recovery than the presence of a focal brain lesion. Mechanical injury to nerve fibers is widespread throughout the brain and is presumed to account for hemispheric disconnection effects.

Injury to the cerebral white matter Holbourn (1943), a physicist, developed a theory about the mechanics of head injury and devised an experimental model to test his formulation of shear strain produced by rotational acceleration. In view of the brain's relative incompressibility as compared to its slight resistance to distortion in shape, Holbourn inferred that rotational acceleration results in shear strain, i.e., pulling apart of axons and disruption of cell bodies. Using a model of colored gelatin within a wax skull (Figure 1-2), he found that shear strains in the gelatin became visible upon sudden forward rotation. He further observed that the greatest shear strain was at the portion of the model corresponding to the anterior tip of the temporal lobe, a finding he explained as a tearing of the brain in this region by the inwardly projecting ridge of the lesser wing of the sphenoid bone. As shown in Figure 1-2, Holbourn's model also provided evidence of lesser shear strains in other parts of the brain. Rotational movement produced shear strain when the head was free to move, but not when it was held in a fixed position.

Holbourn's findings have been confirmed in experimental studies of head injury in animals. Pudenz and Shelden (1946) recorded the movement of the

Fig. 1-2. The effects of violent rotational jerking on a model of the brain constructed of gelatin cast into a paraffin-wax "skull." In addition to prominent shear strains produced in the frontal and temporal lobes of the model after a blow to the occiput, there is a superficial layer of shear strain near the vertex. [From Holbourn, A.H.S. (1943). Mechanics of head injuries. *Lancet,* 2:438–441. Reproduced with permission from the publisher.]

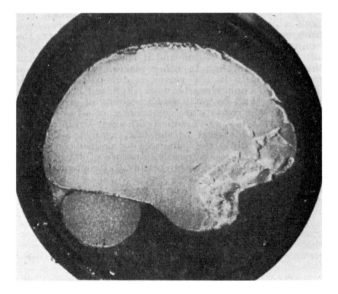

brain during impact to the head by high speed cinematography, using monkeys whose calvariums had been replaced by transparent covers. They observed swirling and gliding movements of the brain when the head was free to move.

Holbourn's contention that shear strains are greater in the areas of the brain characterized by structural irregularity (e.g., temporal lobes) has received support from subsequent experimental head injury studies. Ommaya and Gennarelli (1974) reported that diffuse injury produced by shear strain was greater in areas of bony protrusion (e.g., the tip of the temporal lobe) and rough surfaces (e.g., the frontal pole). In contrast, shear strain was found to be slight in areas of smooth surfaces, such as the occipital lobe. From Holbourn's theoretic analysis and observations of a physical model subjected to rotation and the results of their experimental studies on animals, Ommaya and Gennarelli proposed that the distribution of damage in shear strains "would decrease in magnitude from the surface to the center of the approximately spheroidal brain mass." They postulated that there is "increasing severity of disturbance in level and content of consciousness caused by mechanically induced strains affecting the brain in a centripetal sequence of disruptive effect on function and structure." The sequence begins on the surface of the brain in cases of mild closed head injury and extends inward to affect the diencephalic core in the most severe injuries.

Strich (1956) was the first investigator to report pathologic findings from the brains of patients with severe diffuse closed head injuries who had survived for periods from five months to one year while remaining quadraplegic in a profoundly demented or vegetative state. The injuries were presumed to be diffuse because they were not complicated by intracranial hematoma, herniation, or lacerations of the brain. In this series and in a subsequent study of similar injuries (Strich, 1970), she implicated physical damage of nerve fibers at the time of injury and subsequent white matter degeneration as the primary pathologic changes and further pointed out that the brain damage produced by the tearing of nerve fibers at the time of injury is microscopic. Apart from generalized ventricular dilatation (Figure 1-3), which was visualized by antemortem radiologic findings, the only macroscopic brain lesions were seen in the corpus callosum and the superior cerebellar peduncles, in addition to a few cortical contusions and small areas of resolved hemorrhage from torn blood vessels in the cerebral hemispheres. The observed histologic changes (Wallerian degeneration) were the same as those following interruption of axons from other causes.

The disappearance of myelin as cerebral edema resolves contributes to the reduced bulk of cerebral white matter. As shown in Figure 1-4, retraction balls (i.e., beads of axoplasm) form at both ends of an axon within hours of injury.

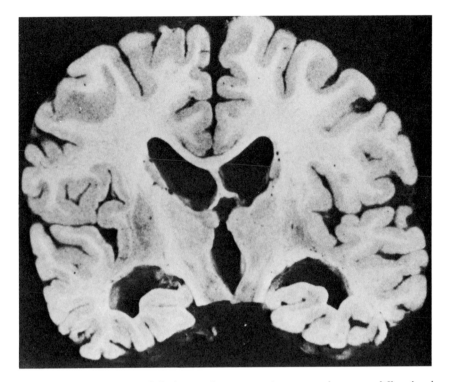

Fig. 1-3. Coronal section of the brain of a patient who sustained a severe diffuse head injury and was rendered comatose immediately after impact. Note the generalized ventricular dilatation and thinning of the corpus callosum. These findings were also common in the injuries studied by Strich (1970). [From Adams, J.H. et al. (1977). Diffuse brain damage of the immediate impact type. *Brain, 100*:489–502. Reproduced with permission of the authors and publisher.]

The retraction ball formed from the portion of the axon severed from the cell body is resorbed within a few weeks, but its proximal end remains visible for months. Figure 1-4 shows numerous retraction balls on a section through the internal capsule of a patient who died after a head injury that produced coma immediately after impact. Strich observed that the frequency of retraction balls was greatest in the corpus callosum, the parasagittal areas of the hemispheres, the internal capsules, and the pons. She also found that the distribution of retractions balls varies with the mechanics of the injury. Bundles of nerve fibers running in one direction may be damaged, whereas nearby bundles running in a different direction may be spared. Degeneration of the white matter was fre-

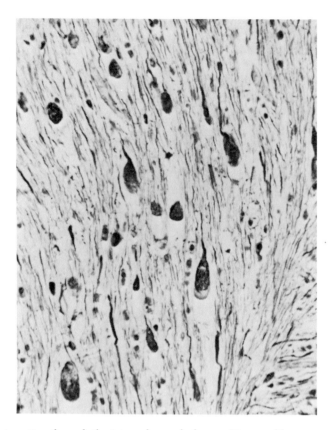

Fig. 1-4. A section through the internal capsule from a 35-year-old woman who died 11 days after a motor vehicle accident without recovering consciousness. Palmgren silver impregnation showed many argyrophilic swellings (retraction balls), some clearly at the ends of ruptured nerve fibers. [From Strich, S.J. (1970). Lesions in the cerebral hemispheres after blunt head injury, in *Pathology of Trauma*. S. Sevitt and H.B. Stoner (eds.). BMA House, London, pp. 166–171. Reproduced with permission of the author and publisher.]

quently asymmetric, anatomic tracts in one hemisphere or on one side of the brain stem being selectively injured.

The pathologic changes described by Strich would have broader implications for neuropsychological recovery from closed head injury if similar effects occurred after less severe head injury. Oppenheimer (1968) has demonstrated lesions of the cerebral white matter in the brains of patients who sustained "mild concussion" and died from complications. In summarizing his findings, he stated that "the point to be stressed in regard to these cases of concussion is that permanent damage, in the form of microscopic destructive foci, can be inflicted on the brain by what are regarded as trivial head injuries."

Neuropathological studies (Adams et al., 1977; Lindenberg et al., 1955; Strich, 1956, 1970) have consistently suggested that in cases of diffuse brain injury there is disproportionately severe damage to the corpus callosum. Figure 1-3, taken from Adams and his coworkers (1977), shows an example of thinning of the corpus callosum in a case of long survival. Lindenberg attributed lesions of the corpus callosum to sudden stretching, as well as to pressure and shearing forces occurring at the moment of impact. The direction of impact was frequently from the vertex to the base of the skull. The extent of the lesions varied from involvement of the entire corpus callosum to small lesions restricted to a circumscribed area. Lindenberg concluded that these lesions are "caused by sudden stretching and shearing forces due to elastic deformation of the skull and brain at the moment of the impact." In all cases, the force was vertically directed.

From a pathologic standpoint, callosal lesions may be divided into hemorrhage, hemorrhage and necrosis, and ischemic necrosis, depending upon the duration of survival and the complications following the injury. Adams, Mitchell, Graham, and Doyle (1977) found macroscopic lesions of the corpus callosum in all cases of diffuse brain injury. They reported that there is frequently a hemorrhagic lesion adjacent to the midline affecting nearly the full thickness of the corpus callosum, extending over a large proportion of the antero-posterior distance of the callosum, and frequently involving the splenium. Histologic examination showed that damage to the corpus callosum extended beyond the hemorrhagic zone insofar as axonal retraction balls (a sign of degenerative changes above and below the level of disruption) were frequently present. In accord with these findings, behavioral evidence of cerebral hemispheric disconnection (e.g., left-sided agraphia, apraxia, and tactile anomia) has been reported after severe head injury (Levin et al., 1981; Rubens et al., 1977; Schott et al., 1969).

Ischemic brain damage   Ischemic hypoxia results when cerebral blood flow (CBF) falls below a critical level. Insofar as cerebral perfusion pressure (i.e., the driving force for cerebral blood flow) is equal to the difference between the mean arterial pressure and intracranial pressure, raised intracranial pressure also contributes to ischemic hypoxia. Other complications of injury (e.g., pulmonary insufficiency) may also contribute to hypoxia. Neuropathological findings suggest that ischemic necrosis is present in about 50% of cases of fatal head injury (Graham and Adams, 1971). Areas of necrosis may include small infarcts at the bottom of sulci or the territory supplied by one of the major arteries. Measurement of regional CBF in head-injured patients with varying degrees of impaired consciousness has supported the concept of ischemic hypoxia. Obrist, Gennarelli, Segawa, Dolinskas, and Langfitt (1979) found that CBF was related to the level of consciousness during the early posttraumatic period and the clinical course. Cerebral blood flow declined markedly in both hemispheres of patients who died or remained vegetative, but progressively increased with neurologic improvement in patients who recovered. In contrast, CBF was above normal (absolute hyperemia) in some patients with CT evidence of acute brain swelling or in patients recovering from profound systemic shock. The finding of hyperemia concomitant with diffuse swelling led Obrist and his coworkers to suggest that increased cerebral blood volume may contribute to compression of the cerebrospinal fluid spaces. This interpretation was supported by measurement of higher density coefficients of the CT scan.

Brain swelling/edema   Brain edema, which results from the accumulation of excess water in the brain tissue, is usually found around areas of vascular damage. Traumatic edema is at least initially "vasogenic," i.e., the source of the excess water is leakage of fluid from cerebral blood vessels. Leaking plasma from a cortical contusion can spread to the underlying white matter by passing between the myelin sheaths. Figure 1-5 shows a CT scan of an intracerebral hematoma surrounded by edematous tissue. Depending on the spatial distribution of edema, it may be considered a diffuse process. Apart from contributing to an expanding mass effect, it is uncertain whether edema per se damages the brain.

Computerized tomographic evidence of massive cerebral swelling, i.e., a generalized increase in brain volume, is common in young patients within 24 hours of severe head injury (but can occur in older patients) and may be detected as early as one-half hour after injury (Kobrine, Timmins, Rajjoub, Rizzoli, and Davis, 1977). Diffuse cerebral swelling is thought to result from hyperemia, i.e., cerebral blood flow in excess of the metabolic needs of the brain. Obrist and his coworkers describe this condition as "relative hyperemia" when the absolute level of cerebral blood flow in head-injured patients remains within normal limits as compared to control subjects. The ventricles and cisterns appear compressed or obliterated (Figure 1-6A) and a slight elevation of brain CT density values (consistent with cerebrovascular engorgement) imparts a homogeneous gray appearance to the white matter. Follow-up CT (Figure 1-6B) frequently shows recovery of the ventricles to at least normal size and a decline in density

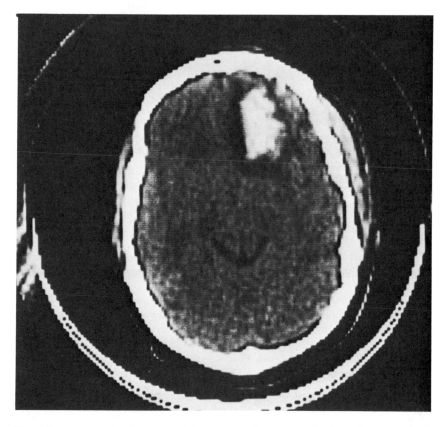

Fig. 1-5. Computerized tomographic scan visualizing a right frontal intracerebral hematoma surrounded by a ring of decreased density indicating edema. The CT scan was performed four days after a head injury sustained in a motor vehicle accident.

values of the white matter. A consecutive series of severe closed head-injury admissions without acute intracranial hematoma admitted to the Institute of Neurological Sciences in Glasgow showed CT evidence of generalized brain swelling in more than one-third of the patients (Snoek et al., 1979). Pathologic findings in the fatal cases disclosed diffuse white matter injury, hypoxic cortical damage, cerebral contusion, and signs of increased intracranial pressure. The authors cautioned that diffuse white matter injury in these cases was discernible only at a microscopic level and thus could not be appreciated by CT.

The CT pattern of generalized brain swelling is particularly frequent after head injury in children (Figure 1-6A,B). Zimmerman, Bilaniuk, Bruce, Dolin-

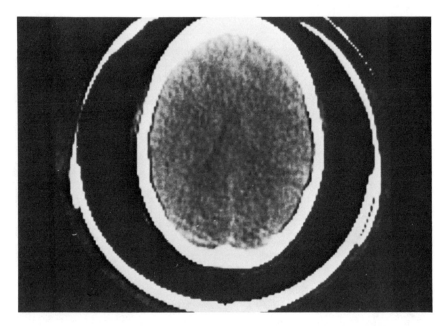

Fig. 1-6A. Computerized tomographic scan obtained on the day of injury in a 23-year-old woman who sustained a closed head injury in a motor vehicle accident. Generalized brain swelling is suggested by the obscuration of the lateral ventricles.

Fig. 1-6B. Followup CT scan performed one-month postinjury in the same patient showing enlargement of the ventricles to within the limits of normal variation.

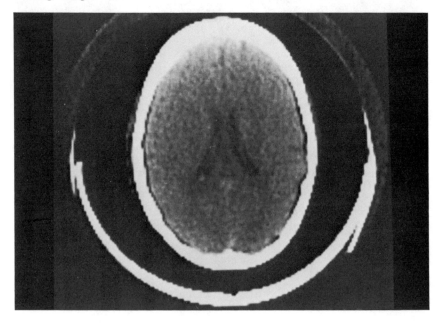

skas, Obrist, and Kuhl (1978) reported that more than one-quarter of a consecutive series of pediatric closed head injury admissions exhibited this finding on the initial CT scan, which was obtained within 24 hours of injury in most cases. On the basis of their recordings of regional cerebral blood flow, the authors attributed the cerebral swelling to transitory hyperemia rather than to edema.

Secondary insult to the injured brain   The severity of brain damage after serious head injury can be increased by systemic complications arising immediately after injury, during emergency evacuation, or after arrival in the emergency room. In a consecutive series of severe closed head injury admissions, Miller, Sweet, Narayan, and Becker (1978) found that almost one-half of the group suffered from one or more systemic complications, such as hypotension, anemia, hypoxia, or hypercarbia, at the time of admission. These systemic complications were most common in head-injured patients with multiple injuries (e.g., long bone fracture or a pelvic fracture). Systemic complications were associated with a poorer outcome in patients with diffuse closed head injuries, most of whom were injured in moving vehicle accidents. In contrast, their presence did not alter the outcome of severe closed head injury complicated by a mass lesion.

Intracranial pressure

The intracranial space may be viewed as a rigid container, the compartments of which are blood, brain, and cerebrospinal fluid. Within limits, the intracranial pressure is maintained at a constant level despite volumetric changes in one or another of the intracranial components (e.g., blood). When the volume of one component is increased, an equal volume of one of the other components is displaced. Measurement of the pressure-volume relationship within the cranium yields an exponential curve (Figure 1-7) in which an initial flat portion is followed by a steeper segment. The initial flat portion of a curve is generally attributed to displacement of cerebrospinal fluid and blood from the cranial cavities, whereas the steep segment of the curve is reached when cerebrospinal fluid buffering is exhausted and the elastic properties of brain and blood predominate. Provided that no permanent increase in the volume of one compartment occurs, intracranial pressure is held constant.

Elevated intracranial pressure (20 mm Hg or greater) occurs in more than 75% of patients with severe closed head injury, and it is often associated with an intracranial hematoma or generalized cerebral swelling (Miller et al., 1977).

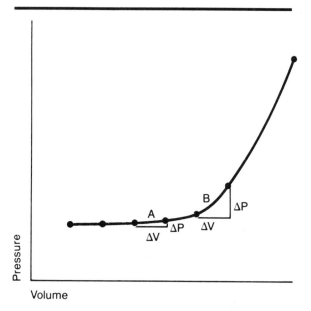

Fig. 1-7. Intracranial pressure plotted against intracranial volume. Experimental studies demonstrated that the pressure-volume relationship is represented by an exponential curve in which an initial flat portion is followed by a steeper segment. [From Bruce, D.A. (1978). The Pathophysiology of Increased Intracranial Pressure. *Current Concepts.* The Upjohn Company, p. 19. Reproduced with permission of the author and publisher.]

Uncontrolled intracranial pressure frequently causes diffuse ischemic brain damage and probably accounts for close to 50% of the mortality after closed head injury (Bakay and Glasauer, 1980). A potentially serious elevation of intracranial pressure occurs during a plateau wave that frequently starts from a normal baseline and rises to high pressures for 5 to 20 minutes. The rise in pressure is produced by cerebral vasodilatation.

Neurologic intensive care units frequently employ continuous recording of intracranial pressure through a catheter placed in the lateral ventricle. The output is connected to a strain gauge and pressure transducer, which is traced on a paper chart recorder. Insertion of a subarachnoid bolt connected to a strain gauge and recorder is an alternate method of continuous pressure recording. Monitoring intracranial pressure may alert the neurosurgeon to the threat of herniation.

Relationship between intracranial pressure and brain herniation

After the point is passed on the pressure-volume curve when the buffering capacity of cerebrospinal fluid is exhausted, further increases in volume by hyperemia or an expanding mass lesion may create a large pressure difference between the cerebral compartments and thus cause herniation. The most common type after head injury is transtentorial or uncal herniation, which may result from a supratentorial mass lesion or by diffuse swelling. Transtentorial herniation is characterized by downward displacement of the parahippocampal gyrus and uncus of one or both temporal lobes through the tentorial hiatus. Midbrain injury is frequently secondary to transtentorial herniation of the medial aspect of the hippocampal gyrus or swelling of the temporal lobe. Lateral dislocation of the brain stem thrusts the midbrain against the tentorial margin. Compression and distortion of the midbrain and pons may also result in hemorrhage and structural damage of these structures. The clinical signs are decreased level of consciousness, dilatation and loss of the light reaction of the ipsilateral pupil because of compression of the third nerve, and hemiparesis on the opposite side because of compression of the cerebral peduncle. Unchecked herniation produces deterioration in brain stem functioning, which is often reflected in respiratory abnormality, hyperventilation, decerebration, and eventually, death. Herniation of the cerebellum through the foramen magnum is characterized by symptoms related to compression of the vagus nucleus, hypoxia, and edema of the medulla. Although a shift of midline brain structures may occur with normal intracranial pressure, transtentorial herniation is closely associated with raised pressure.

Focal lesions

The neuropsychological significance of lateralized mass lesions in closed head injury patients is generally less impressive than the findings reported in cases of circumscribed missile injury of the brain (Newcombe, 1969). As described in the following chapters, however, the study of focal lesions in closed head injury patients by CT has disclosed evidence of specific neuropsychological deficit (cf. Uzzell, Zimmerman, Dolinskas, and Obrist, 1979). The major types of focal brain lesion produced by closed head injuries are contusions and intracranial hematomas. Although a delimited area of edema may contribute to mass effect, its margins are usually not as clearly defined as in contusions and hematomas.

Contusion   Transient distortion and inbending of the skull near the point of impact may result in a cerebral contusion. Contusions are also produced by sudden "dislocation of the brain," i.e., when it is thrust against or compressed by a portion of the skull (Courville, 1945). Coup contusion is one under the area of impact, whereas a contrecoup contusion is located at a distance from the point of impact. Gurdjian and Gurdjian (1976) state that contrecoup contusions result from relative movement of the brain during impact. They classify frontotemporal surface contusions after frontal or occipital impact as contrecoup because these result from movement of the brain against the bony irregularities at the base of the skull. Similarly, the Gurdjians suggest that the dural extensions into the cranial cavity forming the falx cerebri and tentorium contribute to contusions on the medial surface of the hemispheres and the corpus callosum injury. In contrast, occipital contrecoup contusions are less frequent because the skull cavity is relatively smooth.

Contusional injuries have a varied appearance on CT. Lanksch, Grumme, and Kazner (1979) differentiate three types of brain contusion visualized by CT. The first appears as a circumscribed area of decreased density, which occurs most frequently in the white matter, and is usually attributed to edema. Focal neurologic signs may accompany this type of contusion. In contrast to this lesion, the second type of contusion has a mottled appearance representing small punctate hemorrhages (areas of increased density) intermixed with normal or edematous (patches of decreased density) brain tissue. This type of contusion is illustrated in Figure 1-8. Zimmerman, Bilaniuk, Dolinskas, Genneralli, Bruce, and Uzzell (1977), who referred to this lesion as an intracerebral hemorrhagic contusion, found it to be the most frequent parenchymal abnormality visualized by CT in head-injured patients. The degree of heterogeneity in density varies as does the presence of perifocal edema, shown by an area of decreased density surrounding the lesion. In general, the hemorrhagic component of a contusion is most clearly visualized as a zone of increased density within two days of injury, whereas the areas of decreased density persist (Zimmerman et al., 1977).

The third type of contusion differentiated by Lanksch, Grumme, and Kazner is bilateral and is presumably caused by coup–contrecoup injury. The authors surmised that a force vector at right angles to the sagittal plane, or in a diagonal plane, is responsible for this type of lesion.

Laceration involves tearing of the surface of the brain and the overlying leptomeninges. These lesions are more likely to be epileptogenic than contusions (Jennett, 1979) and are often surrounded by a larger zone of edema. Subarachnoid blood or formation of a subdural hematoma may result from a laceration because of oozing from the injured blood vessels.

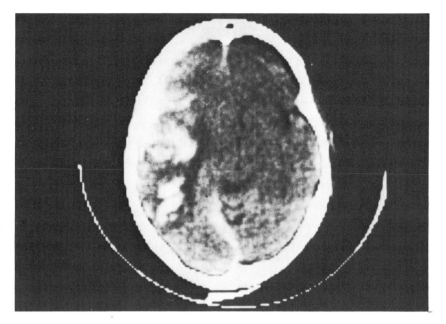

Fig. 1-8. Computerized tomographic scan obtained on the day of injury showing a massive area of contusion in the left parietal region extending into the left frontal and temporal areas. The lateral ventricle on the left is obliterated and midline structures are shifted toward the right. There was also a small left tentorial subdural hematoma. The mottled appearance of this scan conforms to the Type II contusion of Lanksch, Grumme, and Kazner (1979).

Intracranial hematoma   Intracranial hematomas, i.e., space-occupying clots, are found in about 15% of brains examined after fatal head injury (Strich, 1969) and in 30% to 40% of consecutive admissions for severe closed head injury to university hospitals (cf. Miller et al., 1981). Microscopic hemorrhages, which commonly accompany macroscopic hematomas, are formed by shearing forces that tear blood vessels at the time of impact (Strich, 1970). The subcortical white matter and the corpus callosum are frequent sites of parenchymal hemorrhage. Brain stem hemorrhage may also occur. Similar in anatomic distribution to contusions, hematomas are common in the orbital surface of the frontal lobe and the temporal lobe. Intracranial hematomas are classified according to their anatomic sites.

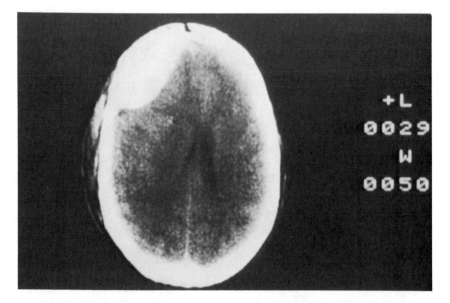

Fig. 1-9. Acute left frontal epidural hematoma appearing in the CT scan as a biconvex zone of increased density adjacent to the calvarium. Note the shift and obliteration of the left lateral ventricle reflecting the mass effect of the hematoma.

Extradural hematoma Extradural hematoma occurs between the skull and the dura. Acute epidural hematomas often appear in the CT scan as biconcave zones of increased density adjacent to the calvarium (Figure 1-9). Epidural hematomas tend to spread in a cranio-caudal direction and thus appear in several slices of the CT scan. An epidural hematoma may appear as an area of mixed density when it contains freshly coagulated and as yet uncoagulated fluid (hypodense). Large epidural hematomas may produce contralateral shift of midline structures and the lateral ventricles as a result of tentorial herniation of the temporal lobe.

Subdural hematoma A subdural hematoma, i.e., a collection of blood between the dura and the arachnoid, results from damage to arteries and veins in injured cortical tissue. In addition, subdural hematomas can arise from a tear in veins extending from the surface of the brain to the dura or from injury to a sinus or to an artery on the surface of the brain. Tearing of the bridging veins of the sagittal sinus is a common etiology for acute subdural hematomas. Subdural hematomas are classified according to their time of onset in relation to the initial injury. An acute subdural hematoma typically requires surgical evacuation within 24 hours of injury, whereas if it develops within two to ten days after injury, it would be considered subacute. A chronic subdural hematoma, which may develop after an apparently trivial injury, can result in symptoms that first appear weeks or months after injury. Chronic subdural hematomas are more common in the elderly, in whom accumulation of blood is facilitated by cerebral atrophy.

Computerized tomographic findings in an acute subdural hematoma show fresh blood in the subdural space as a white band (increased density) conforming to the convex surface of the underlying cerebral hemisphere (Figure 1-10). Zones of normal or decreased density may appear within the total area of the lesion. Over the course of several weeks after evacuation of an acute or subacute

Fig. 1-10. Acute right parietal subdural hematoma appearing as a thin band of increased density over the right hemisphere in a CT scan performed on the day of injury. This 23-year-old man was injured in a motor vehicle accident.

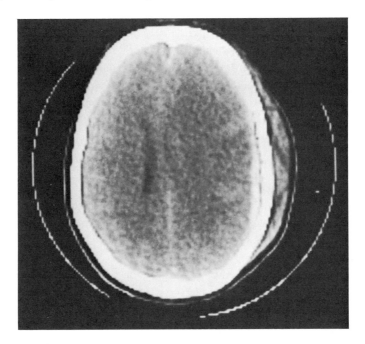

hematoma, the brain tissue undergoes a reduction in tissue density. Although more chronic subdural hematomas may escape detection by CT because their density is similar to adjacent brain tissue, scanning after intravenous administration of a contrast media may enhance detection. The presence of an isodense subdural hematoma may also be suspected from a contralateral shift of the septum pellucidum, third ventricle, and pineal body or from an ipsilateral ventricular compression with enlargement of the contralateral ventricle.

Subdural hygroma   This is a collection of cerebrospinal fluid in the subdural space through a tear in the arachnoid membrane. Subdural hygroma, which has the same density as cerebrospinal fluid, appears under the skull vault and develops within days or weeks after injury. A subdural hygroma may form after the evacuation of an acute subdural hematoma (Lanksch et al., 1979).

Intracerebral hematoma   This is an accumulation of blood within the brain parenchyma, which varies considerably in size. In contrast to a hemorrhagic contusion, an intracerebral hematoma appears on the CT scan as an area of homogeneous high density, which resolves slowly (Figure 1-11). A lucent ring, presumed to reflect edema, develops around a resolving intracerebral hematoma (Zimmerman et al., 1977). There is evidence to suggest that intracerebral hemorrhage of the basal ganglia is particularly likely to occur after closed head injury in children as a result of injury to the lateral branch of the perforator of the middle cerebral artery (Maki, Akimoto, and Enomoto, 1980). Hemorrhage in the basal ganglia frequently produces a contralateral hemiparesis. A case of a left hemisphere intracerebral hematoma involving the putamen and the posterior limb of the internal capsule is shown in Figure 1-11. This 12-year-old, left-handed girl developed a right hemiparesis and was mute for 16 days after injury.

Traumatic subarachnoid and intraventricular hemorrhage   Hemorrhage into the ventricle traditionally has been regarded as a grave prognostic sign. However, CT findings indicate that ventricular hemorrhage occurs more frequently than had been previously thought and that this type of injury does not necessarily have a fatal outcome (Lanksch et al., 1979).

   Traumatic subarachnoid hemorrhage is produced by injury to blood vessels in the pia mater. Severe bleeding into the cerebrospinal fluid spaces appears as an area of increased density on the CT scan. Subarachnoid hemorrhage is usually associated with contusional injury and acute subdural hematoma, frequently in the region of the basal cisterns, in the Sylvian fissure and the sulci

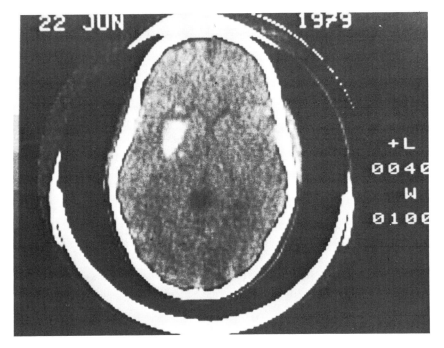

Fig. 1-11. Left hemisphere intracerebral hematoma involving the putamen and the posterior limb of the internal capsule of a 12-year-old girl who was struck by a car. The CT scan was obtained within an hour of injury.

(Lanksch et al., 1979). Subarachnoid bleeding may obstruct the passage of cerebrospinal fluid over the surface of the brain and prevent its absorption.

Hypothalamic–pituitary lesions

Injury to the hypothalamic–pituitary axis may complicate neurobehavioral recovery from closed head injury because of persistent depression, disproportionate psychomotor retardation, and diminished sexual function. Diabetes insipidus is a widely recognized sequel of closed head injury, and signs of hypopituitism have also been described (Crompton, 1971b; Paxson and Brown, 1976). Pathologic evidence suggests that high velocity injuries produce shearing forces that disrupt the hypothalamic neurohypophyseal pathways, leading to abnormal secretion of antidiuretic hormone (Paxson and Brown, 1976). Crompton inferred that lesions of the hypothalamic supraoptic nuclei and infundibulum may produce diabetes insipidus, in a way similar to stalk transection, by denervating the posterior lobe of the pituitary. Commenting upon a tendency for hypothalamic and pituitary lesions to occur together in the same cases, Crompton surmised that damage to the pituitary stalk and perforating vessels to the hypothalamus results from movement of the brain within the skull. He found that hypothalamic lesions were associated with infarction or hemorrhage in the pituitary and inferred that the principal site of injury was in the lower hypothalamus, the infundibulum, and the upper half of the stalk.

The impression from pathologic evidence that posttraumatic diabetes insipidus is primarily attributable to damage to the pituitary stalk or hypothalamic centers (cf. Daniel and Treip, 1966) has received support from neuroendocrine investigations of head-injured patients with prolonged coma (Fleischer et al., 1978). Hypothyroidism and hypogonadism were present within a week after a head injury that produced coma lasting longer than two weeks. Recovery from endocrine defects generally paralleled an improved level of consciousness. From the results of provocative tests with releasing hormones, the authors inferred that the posttraumatic endocrine defects were of suprahypophyseal origin. Girard and Marelli (1977) reported a case of posttraumatic hypothalamic–pituitary insufficiency in a prepubertal boy in whom growth retardation appeared soon after recovery from a severe head injury.

In summary, the shearing forces implicated in producing lesions of the cranial nerves are probably also responsible for damage to the hypothalamic–pituitary system. There is evidence that subclinical, or at least transient endocrine disturbance may be a frequent effect of severe head injury.

Cranial nerve injury

The effects of cranial nerve injury bear on the quality of outcome because of the limitations imposed by sensory loss. Moreover, it is necessary to distinguish nonaphasic disturbance of speech (e.g., dysphonia) related to involvement of the lower cranial nerves from that related to hemispheral injury. Russell (1960) reviewed the cranial nerve findings in 1,000 cases of blunt accidental head injury who were treated at the Oxford Head Injury Hospital during World War II.

Olfactory nerve   Four percent of the patients had complete bilateral anosmia, and in an additional 3%, there was unilateral anosmia or some diminution of the sense of smell. Russell also reported that 12 patients experienced a perversion of the sense of smell. He implicated fracture of the cribiform plate in patients sustaining a frontal impact as well as tearing of the olfactory filaments by shearing movement of the brain relative to the skull.

Optic nerve   Russell implicated frontal impact in producing injury to the optic nerve, which he estimated to occur in 2% of all closed head injury patients. He noted that the severity of visual loss could range from diminished acuity to complete blindness. Russell also pointed out that visual loss after closed head injury may result from occipital lobe contusion. Necropsy findings have most frequently shown ischemic necrosis and shearing injury of the optic foramen and intracranial optic nerve (Crompton, 1970).

Optic chiasm   Chiasmal injury produces visual field defects ranging from unilateral blindness combined with contralateral temporal field depression to a variety of other bitemporal hemianopic defects (Savino et al., 1980). In reviewing the Oxford series, Russell reported that injury to the optic chiasm was rare (0.2%) and was usually a result of frontal impact accompanied by multiple cranial fractures. He suggested that a stretch lesion with tearing of the chiasm was an important mechanism of injury, although contusion hemorrhage and necrosis may be contributory. Savino, Glaser, and Schatz (1980) reported that chiasmal injury was, however, compatible with a wide range of closed head injuries.

Oculomotor lesion   Russell reported that palsies of the third, fourth, or sixth cranial nerves occur in about 3% of accidental head injury cases who survive and observed that injury to these nerves could occur either alone or in combination. In contrast to injuries to the olfactory and optic nerves, Russell found that lesions of the oculomotor nerves were resolved within two to three months of injury and that a variety of oculomotor disorder may occur after injury.

Trigeminal nerve   In Russell's study, injury to the supraorbital branch of the trigeminal was the most common type of trigeminal injury. A scalp wound, or an injury to the upper margin of the orbit, was frequently responsible.

Facial nerve   Injury to the facial nerve causes paralysis of the facial muscles on the same side, frequently resulting in a nonaphasic speech disturbance. Facial paralysis followed closed head injury in about 3% of the patients reviewed by Russell. Fracture of the petrous part of the temporal bone was frequently responsible, unless it was associated with hemorrhage into the middle ear. Russell noted that patients were divided nearly equally between those who have immediate and those who have delayed facial nerve injury.

Eighth nerve   Impairment of hearing in one or both ears was found in 8% of the Oxford head-injury series. Fracture of the middle fossa of the skull was the most frequent cause. True vertigo, which may follow closed head injury is probably due to diffuse injury of or hemorrhage into the labyrinth. Movement of the head or eyes may bring on a violent feeling of unsteadiness, with apparent motion of objects, as well as possible nausea or vomiting.

Cranial nerves IX–XII   Fracture of the base of the skull may result in injury to cranial nerves IX–XII. Fracture of the base of the posterior fossa may result from falls on either the crown of the head or the feet. Involvement of the glossopharyngeal nerve may produce difficulty in swallowing, loss of taste on the posterior one-third of the tongue, and paralysis of some of the pharyngeal muscles. Injury to the vagus nerve may result in paralysis of one side of the palate or of one vocal cord. Damage to the spinal accessory nerve may result in paralysis of the sternomastoid muscle and weakness of the trapezius muscle. Injury of the hypoglossal nerve may result in wasting and paralysis of one-half the tongue, so that on protrusion it deviates to the weak side.

Injury to the skull

Impact causes the skull to undergo deformation. About 75% of human fractures are linear, whereas 25% are depressed or comminuted. Bone fragments in a depressed skull fracture may result in laceration of the underlying brain, producing a focal cortical lesion that is potentially epileptogenic. A linear skull fracture is caused by elastic deformation of the skull. The area of impact is bent in, while the surrounding skull is bent out. Tears of venous sinuses and meningeal vessels may be associated with linear and depressed skull fracture.

A fracture across the middle meningeal groove or over the sagittal sinus may produce an extradural hematoma. A fracture running across the anterior fossa may produce cerebrospinal fluid rhinorrhea, infection, and, possibly, damage to the olfactory or optic nerves. Fracture of the posterior fossa may produce perforation of the eardrum and bleeding from the external auditory meatus. This injury may also be associated with a facial nerve palsy, cerebrospinal fluid rhinorrhea, injury to the trigeminal nerve, infection, and vertigo. Fracture lines radiate from the impact point and often extend into the base of the skull and connect with the cranial foramina.

Assessment of severity of head injury

The measurement of coma

Depth and duration of coma have long been viewed as the most useful indicants of brain damage. Prior to the development of scales to assess coma, clinicians rated unconsciousness by qualitative distinctions that were inferential, such as "purposeful" and "voluntary," and interpreted an abnormal motor response (e.g., "decorticate") as evidence for an anatomic level of lesion. Wakefulness has generally been inferred from the presence of eye opening and speech, although these criteria are not infallible. Persistently vegetative patients may exhibit sleep-wake cycles, whereas mutistic patients can demonstrate otherwise normal consciousness. Consequently, there is a need to rate each response separately.

To characterize the continuum of coma by a practical and reliable procedure, Teasdale and Jennett (1974) developed the Glasgow Coma Scale (Table 1-2), which evaluates three components of wakefulness independently of each other. The stimulus required to induce eye opening; the best motor response; and the best verbal response. Each type of behavior is described in terms of a well-defined gradient of responses that indicates degrees of increasing dysfunction. According to the proposed criteria, coma is defined as the absence of eye opening, inability to obey commands, and failure to utter recognizable words. This definition corresponds to a total Glasgow Coma Scale score of 8 or less.

The composite Glasgow Coma Scale score ($E + M + V$ or "EMV") has gained wide acceptance as an indicant of the overall severity of head injury. As shown in Figure 1-12, the best response on each component of the Scale is recorded at regular intervals to provide a visual profile of the patient's progress. Although neurosurgeons and neurosurgical nurses achieve a high level of agreement in rating each component of the Glasgow Coma Scale, nearly one out of five observers typically disagree with the opinion of the others (disagreement rate = 0.19) in making the global distinction between "consciousness" and "unconsciousness" (Teasdale, Knill-Jones, and Van Der Sande, 1978). Similarly, the judgment of a "purposeful" motor response is less consistent than ratings of the best motor response on the Glasgow Scale.

The criterion of a Glasgow Coma Scale score of 8 or less is useful for selection of patients with severe closed head injury, but it excludes the majority of head-injured patients who may nevertheless show significant sequelae. Clifton, Grossman, Makela, Miner, Handel, and Sadhu (1980) found a U-shaped distribution of Glasgow Coma Scale scores in 558 patients admitted to university hospitals in Houston and Galveston. Figure 1-13 shows that 53% of all injuries had initial

Table 1-2. The Glasgow Coma Scale°

		Eye opening
None	1	Not attributable to ocular swelling
To Pain	2	Pain stimulus is applied to chest or limbs
To Speech	3	Nonspecific response to speech or shout, does not imply the patient obeys command to open eyes
Spontaneous	4	Eyes are open, but this does not imply intact awareness
		Motor response
No Response	1	Flaccid
Extension	2	"Decerebrate." Adduction, internal rotation of shoulder, and pronation of the forearm
Abnormal Flexion	3	"Decorticate." Abnormal flexion, adduction of the shoulder
Withdrawal	4	Normal flexor response; withdraws from pain stimulus with abduction of the shoulder
Localizes Pain	5	Pain stimulus applied to supraocular region or fingertip causes limb to move so as to attempt to remove it
Obeys Commands	6	Follows simple commands
		Verbal response
No Response	1	(Self-explanatory)
Incomprehensible	2	Moaning and groaning, but no recognizable words
Inappropriate	3	Intelligible speech (e.g., shouting or swearing), but no sustained or coherent conversation
Confused	4	Patient responds to questions in a conversational manner, but the responses indicate varying degrees of disorientation and confusion
Oriented	5	Normal orientation to time, place, and person

Summed Glasgow Coma Scale Score = E + M + V (3 to 15).

°After Teasdale, G., and Jennett, B. (1974). The Glasgow Coma Scale. *Lancet,* 2:81–84.

scores of 13 to 14 (least severe) at the time of admission. In contrast, only 30% of the patients had Glasgow Coma Scale scores of 8 or less (most severe) at the time of admission. Thus, only 17% of the patients had Glasgow Coma Scale scores of 9-12 compatible with head injury of intermediate severity.

In practice, plotting the Glasgow Scale scores at regular intervals serves to identify the neurologic course of patients with acute head injury and yields more useful prognostic information than the scores at the time of admission (Jennett, Teasdale, Braakman, Minderhoud, Heiden, and Kurze, 1979). In a study of 53 head-injured patients who had a Glasgow Coma Scale score of 8 or less for at least six hours, Clifton and his colleagues (1980) identified four distinct patterns of early neurologic course. The first was one of rapid, early improvement in which the rise in coma score was at least four points in the first 48 hours after injury. The second pattern was one of slow improvement, i.e., a rise in

24 HR. NEURO-VITAL FUNCTION

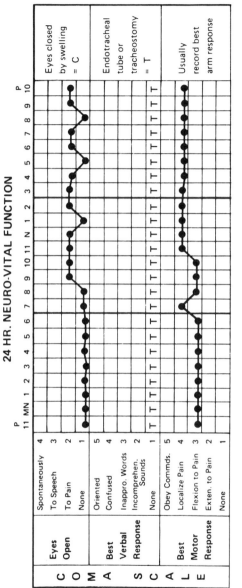

			P 11 MN 1 2 3 4 5 6 7 8 9 10 11 N 1 2 3 4 5 6 7 8 9 P 10	
C O	Eyes Open	Spontaneously	4	Eyes closed by swelling = C
		To Speech	3	
		To Pain	2	
		None	1	
M A S C	Best Verbal Response	Oriented	5	Endotracheal tube or tracheostomy = T
		Confused	4	
		Inappro. Words	3	
		Incomprehen. Sounds	2	
		None	1	
A L E	Best Motor Response	Obey Commds.	5	Usually record best arm response
		Localize Pain	4	
		Flexion to Pain	3	
		Exten. to Pain	2	
		None	1	

Fig. 1-12. Chart showing serial Glasgow Coma Scale scores entered hourly. The "T" indicates that an endotracheal tube was inserted.

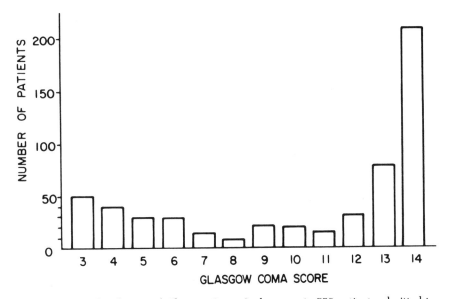

Fig. 1-13. The distribution of Glasgow Coma Scale scores in 558 patients admitted to university hospitals in Houston and Galveston. [From Clifton, G.L., et al. (1980). Neurologic course and correlated computed tomographic findings after severe closed head injury. *J. Neurosurg. 52*:611–624. Reproduced with permission of the authors and publisher.]

coma score of only one or two points within four days of injury. The third pattern consisted of no change in the first week, and the fourth pattern was one of the onset of deterioration after 48 hours. The authors found that death within 48 hours of injury was strongly associated with low initial Glasgow Coma Scale scores (mostly below 6), whereas delayed deterioration was more closely related to the presence of an intracranial hematoma than to the score on the Glasgow Scale. They concluded that "heterogeneity of clinical course and brain pathology make the initial Glasgow Coma Scale score, or that in the first six hours, an incomplete index of severity of injury when series of patients are being compared."

Limitations of the Glasgow Coma Scale Constraints on the administration of the Glasgow Coma Scale include ocular swelling that prevents eye opening and insertion of an endotracheal tube that precludes a verbal response. The use of barbituates and paralytic drugs to lower intracranial pressure (Rockoff, Marshall, and Shapiro, 1979) immobilizes the patient. The Scale is feasible for use only when barbituate therapy is given intermittently. In view of these constraints, the duration of posttraumatic amnesia (described in Chapter 4) may be particularly useful in the assessment of these cases.

The evolution of prolonged coma

The evolution of prolonged coma (greater than two weeks) in 135 patients with severe closed head injury was described by Bricolo, Turazzi, and Feriotti (1980). As shown in Figure 1-14, it was found that restoration of spontaneous or stimulated opening of the eyes occurs in the majority of patients from one to four weeks after injury and in nearly three-fourths of patients by the end of the first month. Restoration of an observable sleep-wake cycle was found in a progressively increasing number of patients over the first six months. When the time-course of recovery was considered in relation to outcome at the end of one year, the return of the capacity to obey simple commands was considered to mark the end of unconsciousness. Most patients who eventually obeyed commands were able to do so within three months after injury (Figure 1-14). Only rarely did a patient recover this capacity after one year.

Figure 1-14 shows that the time of restoration of speech was more variable, the peak period being between three and six months. Very few (1.5%) patients

Fig. 1-14. Stages of recovery from coma persisting longer than two weeks in 135 patients in a follow-up one year after injury. The time-course of restoration of eye opening, obeying commands, and speech is shown. [From Bricolo, A. et al. (1980). Prolonged posttraumatic unconsciousness. Therapeutic assets and liabilities. *J. Neurosurg.* 52:625–634. Reproduced with permission of the authors and publisher.]

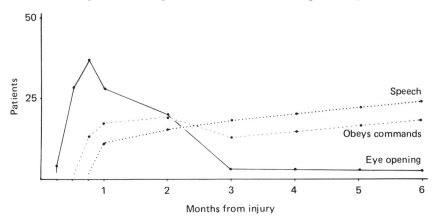

began to talk between the sixth and the twelfth month. At the end of 12 months, there was 30% mortality of the total series, and 8% of the patients remained vegetative. In summary, less than 25% of the patients in this study showed signs of cognitive function within one month after injury, but by three months (and particularly after the sixth month) most patients could no longer be considered to be in coma.

Indicants of brain stem dysfunction

The size and reactivity of the pupils reflect the integrity of the upper brain stem, provided that injury to the third cranial nerve or to the eye itself can be ruled out. An expanding unilateral lesion, which produces herniation with involvement of one side of the midbrain and third nerve, results in dilatation and decreased reactivity of the ipsilateral pupil. Examination of eye movements assesses the integrity of the pathways that pass through both the midbrain and the pons. In patients who are unable to cooperate with testing voluntary eye movements, the vestibular–ocular reflexes are evaluated.

In the comatose patient without direct destruction or compression of the neural pathways controlling eye movements, brisk rotation of the head from one side to the other produces currents in the semicircular canals and, by a reflex mechanism, results in conjugate eye deviation in the opposite direction (e.g., if the head is rotated to the left, the eyes deviate to the right). Similarly, the eyes deviate upward when the neck is flexed and downward when the neck is extended. Impairment of eye movement may occur either because the patient is sufficiently awake to suppress the reflex or because the brain stem is injured. The distinction between these possibilities may be made by testing caloric responses (Figure 1-15).

As shown in Figure 1-15, lateral conjugate eye movements are stimulated by injecting cold water against the tympanic membrane. This is a stronger stimulus for eye movement than passive rotation of the head. If the cortical connections are intact, nystagamus is observed initially. The normal oculovestibular response in the comatose patient is tonic conjugate deviation of both eyes for about one minute toward the irrigated ear followed by a slow return to midline.

Injury to the brain stem often produces abnormal oculocephalic and caloric reflexes that vary with the location of the lesion. In patients with lesions of the third nerve or the medial longitudinal fasciculus, the eye ipsilateral to the lesion fails to adduct to oculocephalic or caloric stimulation. Pontine lesions result in absence of the oculocephalic and caloric responses on the affected side, whereas dorsalateral pontine lesions may produce skew deviation. Although the absence

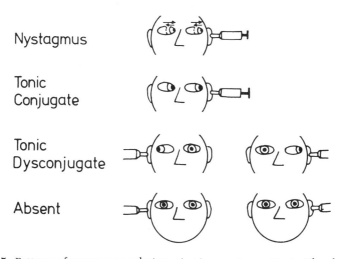

Nystagmus

Tonic
Conjugate

Tonic
Dysconjugate

Absent

Fig. 1-15. Patterns of response to caloric testing in comatose patients. The abnormalities of tonic dysconjugate and absent eye movements are described in the text. [From Teasdale, G. (1976). Assessment of head injuries. *Br. J. Anaesth.* 48:761–766. Reproduced with permission of the author and publisher.]

of the oculovestibular response in the comatose patient is viewed as evidence for brain stem injury, Plum and Posner (1980) note that some types of medication (e.g., barbituates) may block the response.

Prognostic implications of acute neurologic deficit

Investigators have analyzed the indicants of neurologic impairment that are most predictive of global outcome (Braakman et al., 1980; Clifton et al., 1980; Jennett et al., 1976, 1979; Miller et al., 1981). Deterioration leading to death more than 48 hours after injury is associated with delayed development of an intracranial hematoma, the onset of increased hemispheric edema, systemic complications, and a decline in the summed score of the Glasgow Coma Scale during the first week (Clifton et al., 1980).

Predictors of outcome at six months after closed head injury producing coma (no eye opening, failure to obey commands, and inability to utter recognizable words) for at least six hours have been studied in patients whose case histories are stored in an international data bank of severe head injury (Braakman et al., 1980; Jennett et al., l976, 1979; Jennett and Teasdale, 1981). The findings from Glasgow and Rotterdam are in close agreement in their indications that mortality rises exponentially as age of the patient at the time of injury increases. The presence of bilaterally impaired pupillary reaction to light at the time of admission or during the initial month after injury is also a useful predictor of outcome at six months or more postinjury (Braakman et al., 1980; Jennett et al., 1976, 1979; Miller et al., 1981). Consistent with the findings of Clifton and coworkers concerning the early posttraumatic course, the summed score of the Glasgow Coma Scale during the first 24 hours and changes in the score over time are also predictive of outcome at six months postinjury (Braakman et al., 1980; Jennett et al., 1979). During the first week after severe head injury, the motor response is the most powerful predictor of the three components of the Glasgow Coma Scale. Miller and his colleagues (1981) found that the presence of an abnormal motor response (i.e., a score of over 4 on the motor portion) was related to greater mortality, particularly in nonsurgical cases.

Spontaneous eye movements or the interrelated reflex eye movement have been reported to be important prognostic signs (Braakman et al., 1980; Jennett et al., 1976, 1979). However, the results of Braakman et al. have shown that the degree of interobserver agreement for evaluation of spontaneous eye movements and oculocephalic/oculovestibular responses is below the level of agreement for the Glasgow Coma Scale and observation of pupillary reactivity. Although an autonomic abnormality (e.g., pulse over 120/minute) is also associated with a poor outcome after severe closed head injury, Jennett, Teasdale, Braakman, Minderhoud, Heiden, and Kurze (1979) found that this indicant contributes little additional prognostic information beyond that contributed by other predictors.

Miller and his colleagues (1981) have reported that raised intracranial pressure (mean persistently above 20 mm Hg) that could not be controlled was associated with a high mortality. The quality of survival was poor even in cases in whom elevated pressure could be brought under control.

There is evidence to suggest that the patient's level of early activity is related to long-term recovery. Reyes, Bhattacharyya, and Heller (1981) rated the activity level of closed head injury patients after they had emerged from coma (median duration 1.5 weeks) and were transferred to a rehabilitation hospital. The authors found a U-shaped relationship between early posttraumatic activity level and overall improvement, both upon discharge from the rehabilitation hospital and at followup (mean of four years). Patients who either were sluggish or markedly agitated fared worse than patients who were appropriately active or slightly restless after the comatose period.

Adverse neurologic signs may have even greater prognostic significance when they occur in combination. Becker, Miller, Ward, Greenberg, Young, and Sakalas (1977) found that a motor response worse than localizing to pain had grave consequences when it was accompanied by impaired or absent oculocephalic responses and bilateral absence of pupillary reaction to light in that 76% of these patients died. Similarly, the adverse influence of an intracranial hematoma on outcome may be related to the circumstance of being more common in older patients (Jennett et al., 1979).

Neuroradiologic procedures

Computerized tomographic scanning has displaced angiography as the primary procedure to characterize the pathology of acute closed head injury. Serial CT imaging, combined with recording of Glasgow Coma Scale scores and other neurologic findings, is extremely useful in elucidating the early clinical course after severe head injury (Clifton et al., 1980). The characteristic features of CT imaging after closed head injury are summarized in the preceding sections (Mechanisms of diffuse injury and focal lesions) and are described in the section on delayed ventricular enlargement, which follows. For an informative review of CT in head injury, the reader is referred to the book by Lanksch, Grumme, and Kazner (1979).

Plain skull films are used to identify the linear and depressed fractures described in the preceding discussion of the pathology of head injury. In comparison with older radiologic techniques, CT aids in identifying contusions and hematomas associated with depressed skull fractures and in demonstrating soft tissue lesions (e.g., of the paranasal sinus) that frequently complicate injury to the frontal base of the skull. Computerized tomography can visualize a brain abscess which may be a late complication of injury. Both bone and soft tissue lesions of the orbit may also be shown by CT.

Clinical neurophysiologic procedures

Since the CT scan has become widely available, the conventional electroencephalogram (EEG) is less frequently employed in the clinical assessment of acute closed head injury. The EEG, however, is essential to investigate posttraumatic epilepsy (described later in this chapter). Recently developed techniques, including computer analysis of the EEG, evoked cortical and brain stem potentials, event related potentials, and direct stimulation and recording from the cortex, provide information concerning the functional integrity of the brain. Detailed reviews of electrophysiologic findings after head injury have been recently published (Bricolo et al., 1979; Grossman, 1979). Only the most salient findings are summarized here.

Serial EEG tracings recorded during the early phases of recovery from severe closed head injury exhibit slowing of spontaneous electrical activity, often to the 1 to 4 Hz (delta-) range. The normal spatial distribution of rhythms of different frequencies is often lost. The usual findings of fast rhythms frontally and slower (alpha) rhythms posteriorly may be replaced by a relatively uniform rhythm in all leads. Spontaneous fluctuation in the dominant frequency may be reduced and the arousal response to sensory stimulation may be abnormal or completely abolished. In severe injuries, there may be "paradoxical" arousal, a condition in which the typical response to painful stimulation (low voltage fast activity) is replaced by high voltage slow activity.

As a patient recovers from a comatose state, serial EEG recordings typically show a progressive increase in the frequency of the alpha waves, a greater spontaneous variation in frequency, and a more normal responsiveness to stimuli. Employing spectral analysis of the EEG, Steudel and Druger (1979) found that an increase of the amplitude in the theta- and alpha- range during the first week after severe head injury was predictive of survival. Similarities between the EEG of normal sleep and the tracings recorded in comatose patients after severe head injury have been described (cf. Grossman, 1979). Lateralized mass lesion can produce hemispheric asymmetry in the voltage and frequency. Injuries that lacerate or penetrate the cortex produce seizure activity on the EEG in about 50% of the cases.

Sensory-evoked potentials have been shown to be sensitive to head injury. In experimental studies, deterioration in the evoked potential has been found to be related to impairment of consciousness and to reduced cerebral blood flow in primates subjected to rotational acceleration of the head (Ommaya and Gennarelli, 1974). Recovery of the potential and of consciousness occurred in parallel.

Greenberg and his coworkers (1977) have reported the most detailed study of multimodality-evoked potentials in head-injured patients. They classified the degree of loss of complexity in the somatosensory-, visual-, and auditory-evoked potentials of head-injured patients as compared to normative data. The degree of abnormality in the sensory-evoked potential during the first week after severe head injury was found to be positively related to neurologic findings, including the presence of flexor or extensor posturing, the duration of coma, impaired oculocephalic responses, and pupillary abnormality. Greenberg and his colleagues also found that the degree of abnormality in the evoked potential was related to global outcome. Consistent with this finding, Rappaport and coworkers (1977) reported that the grade of evoked potential was positively correlated with disability ratings of closed head injury patients in a rehabilitation program.

The auditory brain stem evoked response consists of low voltage potentials occurring the first 10 msec after an auditory stimulus. Abnormalities in this potential have been shown to reflect the integrity of the brain stem in comatose patients (Seales, Rossiter, and Weinstein, 1979).

Recording directly from the cerebral cortex can provide information concerning the excitability of a focal area. This procedure has not been commonly employed.

Sensory-evoked potentials assess the functional state of projections to the cortex as well as the cerebral cortex. By electrically stimulating and recording from the cortical surface, the integrity of the cerebral cortex itself can be assessed more directly. The direct cortical response can be recorded serially in situations in which intracranial pressure monitoring is also performed. The direct cortical response is sensitive to anoxia and ischemia, declining in amplitude with decreasing cerebral blood flow and disappearing when cerebral blood is about one-third normal (Grossman, 1979). Cyclical change of the excitability of the cortex is demonstrated by abrupt loss of the direct cortical response in edematous contused cortex at the margins of cortical lacerations or intracerebral hematomas (Grossman et al., 1979). This cyclical loss of activity has been found to be predictive of the development of spike discharges recorded from the cortical surface.

The recording of evoked responses during an ongoing cognitive task may elucidate the neurophysiologic correlates of posttraumatic neuropsychological impairment. In view of the characteristic stages of coma and posttraumatic amnesia, it is plausible that distinctive patterns of evoked potentials during cognitive activity may appear as amnesia and confusion are resolved.

Neurochemical analysis

Clinicians have long observed behavior during the subacute phase of recovery from closed head injury that suggests sympathetic hyperactivity. Agitation, combativeness, screaming, hyperventilation, thrashing, and heightened emotionality are behavioral features that suggest neurochemical alteration. Acute psychosis characterized by hallucinations and delusions in head-injured patients with no antecedent psychiatric disorder (see Chapter 9) also suggests neurochemical changes.

This possibility has received preliminary support in two studies. In a small series of head-injured patients with presumed frontotemporal contusion, who were confused (but not comatose) and agitated, Van Woerkom, Teelken, and Minderhoud (1977) found a decrement in cerebrospinal fluid levels of homovanillic acid and 5-hydroxyindoleacetic acid, suggesting a decrease in cerebral serotonergic and dopaminergic activity. Comatose patients with abnormal oculomotor and oculovestibular responses, however, had evidence only of increased serotonergic activity. More recently, Clifton, Zeigler, and Grossman (1980) found that the plasma norepinephrine level was directly related to the Glasgow Coma Scale score at the time of blood sampling. Viewed in perspective, the level of sympathetic activity, as reflected by circulating norephinephrine, was comparable after severe closed head injury to that observed in normal subjects following vigorous exercise.

In view of the neuropathological evidence for diffuse cerebral involvement after closed head injuries of varying severity, it is plausible that further investigation will elucidate neurochemical correlates of posttraumatic behavioral disturbance. Widespread clinical application of these findings awaits the results of further research.

Delayed complications of closed head injury

Cerebral ventricular enlargement

Ventricular enlargement is a frequent sequel of closed head injury (Kishore, Lipper, Miller, Girevendulis, Becker, and Vines, 1978). In 1 to 2% of head trauma cases, ventricular enlargement is secondary to communicating hydrocephalus in which cerebrospinal fluid flow is disturbed by obstructions in the subarachnoid space (Granholm and Svendgaard, 1972). Signs of communicating hydrocephalus include progressive dementia, gait disturbance, and incontinence. Granholm and Svendgaard also observed emotional disturbance (predominantly aggression) in closed head injury patients who had developed communicating hydrocephalus. The presumed mechanism of posttraumatic obstructive hydrocephalus is subarachnoid hemorrhage, which causes the formation of clots and debris in the basal cisterns, fibrosis and adhesion of the meninges, and obstruction of the pathways through which the cerebrospinal fluid is absorbed (Front, Beks, Georganas, Beekhuis, and Penning, 1972). Impaired absorption may also be due to blockage of the arachnoid villi.

Studies of CT scanning in consecutive series of closed head injury cases have shown that ventricular enlargement without signs of communicating hydrocephalus occurs in more that 25% of severe injuries and may be present as early as two weeks postinjury (Kishore et al., 1978). This finding, which is consistent with neuropathologic evidence of ventriculomegaly in patients surviving for various periods with profound dementia (Strich, 1970), has been attributed to a reduction in the bulk of the cerebral white matter, which leads to a reciprocal increase in the volume of the ventricular system (Adams et al., 1977).

Serial CT scanning has frequently disclosed ventricular enlargement months after the initial trauma in young closed head injury patients. Employing the ventricle brain percent ratio (ventricular area/area of intracranial contents) × 100 to characterize the size of the lateral ventricles, Levin, Meyers, Grossman, and Sarwar (1981) found abnormal ventricular enlargement in 75% of their closed head injury series. Cortical atrophy was mild and uncommon. Figure 1-16A shows a marked ventricular enlargement (VBR = 24) present two years after a severe head injury that resulted in prolonged coma. This patient was moderately disabled at the time of the followup CT scan. In contrast, Figure 1-16B depicts a CT scan obtained one year after a severe closed head injury in a young man of similar age who was in a transition from a vegetative state to severe disability at the time of followup.

In a comprehensive investigation of CT indices of posttraumatic cerebral atrophy, Van Dongen and Braakman (1980) obtained scans one to four years after injury in patients who had been in coma (defined as a state in which the patient did not open his eyes, did not utter recognizable words, and did not obey commands) for at least six hours. They found evidence of cerebral atrophy in 86% of the followup CT scans. Supratentorial atrophy was present in nearly three-fourths of the patients, whereas about one-fourth of the cases had evidence of infratentorial atrophy. The presence of infratentorial atrophy, whether it was present alone or in combination with supratentorial atrophy, was particularly common in patients who had been comatose for more than 24 hours.

There is close agreement among the several radiologic studies that the presence and the severity of atrophic changes are related to the quality of overall recovery (Kishore et al., 1978; Van Dongen and Braakman, 1980). Van Dongen and Braakman found that a good recovery from severe closed head injury was related to a normal followup CT scan or to supratentorial atrophy confined to a single hemisphere, whereas infratentorial atrophy was associated with a poorer outcome. Levin, Meyers, Grossman, and Sarwar (1981) also found that the ventricular brain percent ratio was related to residual cognitive impairment. This finding was particularly characteristic of patients who had a prolonged period of coma as a result of a head injury in a high-speed motor vehicle accident.

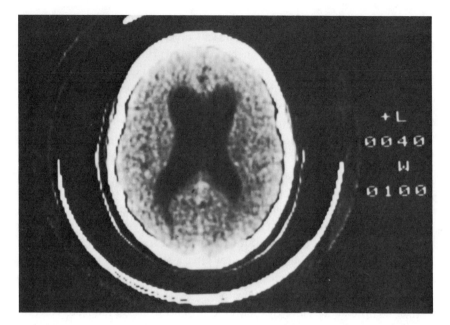

Fig. 1-16A. Computerized tomographic scan performed two years after a severe closed head injury in an 18-year-old student of average preinjury intelligence. Planimetry disclosed a ventricle brain ratio of 24%, more than a fourfold increase above the mean ventricle brain ratio in normal subjects of similar age. The patient recovered to a level of moderate disability characterized by a low normal intellectual ability, severe memory deficit, and inability to maintain employment in a competitive working situation.

Posttraumatic epilepsy

Posttraumatic epilepsy may result from missile injury or closed head injury and appears to arise from areas of brain parenchyma adjacent to scars, cysts, abscess formation, chronic hematomas, and other pathologic sequelae of trauma (Caveness et al., 1979). Although Jennett (1979) found that about 5% of patients developed seizures after civilian closed head injury, the corresponding figure in a recent population study of Olmsted County, Minnesota, was 2% (Annegers et al., 1980). The relative frequency of patients hospitalized for closed head injury who exhibit early epilepsy (within one week of injury and within 24 hours in one-half the cases) is similar to that of patients who develop late seizures that typically occur after three months postinjury (Annegers et al., 1980; Jennett, 1979). In about one-half the early onset cases, the first seizure occurs within 24 hours of injury. Variation in the criteria for hospital admission and case selection

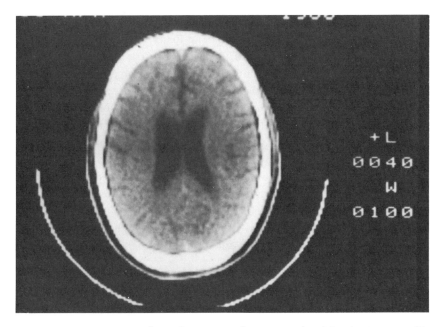

Fig. 1-16B. A CT scan performed one year after severe closed head injury in a 20-year-old man who remained in a vegetative state for nearly one year after injury. He has since improved to the level of severe disability (Chapter 3 provides a description of these categories of outcome). Note the presence of cortical atrophy in addition to ventricular enlargement as compared to the CT scan in Figure 1-16A.

may account for the differences in the relative frequency of posttraumatic epilepsy in the Scottish and American studies.

Focal motor seizures and partial complex ("temporal lobe") seizures predominate in posttraumatic epilepsy. The proportion of patients with posttraumatic seizures after penetrating missile wounds sustained in military action has varied widely across studies (17 to 43%). However, statistics compiled by the National Institutes of Health showed a relatively constant figure of about 33% for American combatants when the statistics from World War I were compared with subsequent wars (Caveness et al., 1979).

Indices of closed head injury associated with greater risk of posttraumatic epilepsy include duration of impaired consciousness (coma, posttraumatic amnesia), focal brain injury associated with a mass lesion or depressed skull fracture, and presence of focal neurologic signs (Jennett, 1979). The most predictive variable of late epilepsy after head injury is the presence of seizures within a week of trauma. Posttraumatic epilepsy after missile wounds of the brain is related to the depth of dural penetration and injury in the region adjacent to the central sulcus (Caveness et al., 1979). The authors commented on the similarity in risk of epilepsy after nonmissile injury complicated by mass lesion or depressed fracture and after missile injury.

Individual differences in susceptibility to posttraumatic seizures are impressive. Children under five years of age are particularly susceptible to early epilepsy. Children who are over two years old when injured are less likely to develop late seizures than are younger children. Caveness and his coworkers (1979) postulated that multifactorial hereditary factors combine with aspects of craniocerebral trauma to determine the likelihood of posttraumatic seizures, their frequency of occurrence, and their persistence. They cited the fairly consistent overall incidence of epilepsy in different wars despite the improvement in neurosurgical management of missile injuries sustained in recent wars as evidence for the role of genetic factors.

Summary

The major mechanism of primary diffuse brain injury after blunt head trauma is mechanical shearing and tearing of nerve fibers and blood vessels. Cerebral swelling and edema also contribute to diffuse injury, although edema can be confined to a circumscribed area. Focal injury, i.e., intracranial hematoma and contusion, is superimposed on a diffuse injury of varying severity. Assessment of the impairment of consciousness provides the most useful quantitative index of the severity of initial injury and the early neurologic course. In combination with the patient's age and pupillary reactivity, the Glasgow Coma Scale has proven to be useful as a predictor of global outcome.

2. Epidemiology

Incidence and prevalence

Incidence and prevalence are the two primary measures of the frequency of a disorder in the community. The incidence of head injury is the number of new cases occurring in a defined population in a specified period of time (usually a year). When the number of new cases is expressed relative to the number of individuals at risk for developing such an injury, an occurrence rate can be calculated. This rate is the probability of a person at risk sustaining a head injury during the designated time period. The prevalence of head injury is the frequency of existing cases, including the number of new cases and all patients from the defined population who survived a previous head injury during a designated time period. Kraus (1980b) specifies further that this measure of morbidity includes only those previous cases of head injury who have not yet recovered, a distinction that may be difficult to make in a survey that does not assess neuropsychological sequelae.

Epidemiologic data for closed head injury in the United States only roughly approximate the actual occurrence of head trauma. Ascertainment of cases is difficult because the International Classification of Diseases (Table 2-1) and other systems of terminology used to code medical records do not reflect current neurosurgical thinking regarding pathophysiology. Further, these systems do not adequately characterize the severity of injury. The reporting of mild injuries treated in emergency rooms is also often incomplete. The admission of patients with mild injuries to a hospital or clinic varies considerably according to geographic factors, outpatient facilities, and patient characteristics (Field, 1976).

Table 2-1. Rubrics for head injury in the International Classification of Diseases°

Fracture of skull

800	Fracture of vault of skull
801	Fracture of base of skull
802	Fracture of face bones
803	Other and unqualified skull fractures
804	Multiple fractures involving skull or face with other bones

Intracranial injury (excluding those with skull fracture)

850	Concussion (differentiates current vs. late effect)
851	Cerebral laceration and contusion
852	Subarachnoid, subdural, and extradural hemorrhage following injury (without mention of laceration or contusion)
853	Other and unspecified intracranial hemorrhage following injury
854	Intracranial injury of other and unspecified nature

Fifth digit subclassification for skull fracture and intracranial injury

0	Unspecified state of consciousness
1	With no loss of consciousness
2	With brief (less than one hour) loss of consciousness
3	With moderate (1 to 24 hours) loss of consciousness
4	With prolonged (more than 24 hours) loss of consciousness and return to preexisting conscious level
5	With prolonged (more than 24 hours) loss of consciousness without return to pre-existing conscious level
6	With loss of consciousness of unspecified duration
9	With concussion, unspecified

°From the Ninth Revision of *The International Classification of Diseases. Clinical Modification. ICD-9-CM.* Vol. 1, Diseases: Tabular List. 1978. Ann Arbor: Edwards Brothers, Inc.

Consequently, there is a lack of uniformity across studies with respect to the inclusion of mild head injury cases.

Field (1976) ascertained the number of cases in England and Wales in 1972 according to his definition of head injury as "trauma which carried some risk of damage to the brain." He confined the collection of data to hospital admissions for patients with predesignated discharge diagnoses. In contrast, the Health Interview Survey sponsored by the National Institute of Neurological and Communicative Disorders and Stroke (NINCDS) in 1975 encompassed cranio-cerebral trauma (including injury to the skull and face without central nervous system involvement) that resulted in at least one day of restricted activity and/or that prompted the patient to seek medical attention (Caveness, 1977; Kraus, 1980a). The inclusion of this variation in the category mild head injury may have contributed to the difference in the estimated incidence of head injury (about 600/100,000 persons in the Health Interview Survey as compared to 430/100,000 persons in Field's study). As expected, these estimates of incidence far exceed the figures obtained in studies in which head injury is defined by a period of unconsciousness or posttraumatic amnesia (Annegers, Grabow, Kurland, and Laws, 1980).

Another requirement for accuracy in a study of incidence is the availability of information about fatally injured patients who die before reaching an emergency room and who may not receive medical attention. These cases account for about 60% of the mortality after head injury (Field, 1976). Most published reports have omitted these patients, resulting in an underestimate of both the occurrence of severe head injury and the case fatality rate. Community incidence studies encompassing a total system of emergency evacuation and treatment within a geographically defined region are in progress in several areas of the United States.

The data reported by Field and by the Health Interview Survey can be compared with the data obtained in Scotland where a centralized system for referring severe injuries facilitated collection. The records of closed head injury patients attending emergency departments throughout the country (population of 4,333,000) for a period of two randomly selected weeks were surveyed by Hawthorne (1978), who reported an incidence of 1,830 cases attending emergency rooms per 100,000 population and hospitalization rate of 322/100,000. Nearly 50% of the admissions were discharged within 24 hours; 7% underwent intracranial surgery.

To assess more accurately the magnitude of the head and spinal cord injury problem in the United States, the NINCDS began the National Head and Spinal Cord Injury (HSCI) Survey in 1974. A detailed description of the method of probability sampling used in this study is provided by Anderson, Kalsbeek, and Hartwell (1980). Briefly, the survey was restricted to hospital admissions for head injury from 1970 to 1974. Consequently, the incidence of severe head injury was underestimated because cases who died before reaching a hospital were excluded. Mild injuries treated in emergency rooms were also excluded. The HSCI Survey employed multistage sampling, which began with a stratified random selection of counties or groups of counties (the primary sampling unit) in the United States from which a sample of hospitals was drawn according to specific criteria. A sample of discharge records was obtained at each hospital for a predetermined portion of the time interval of 1970 through 1974. To be included in the discharge sample, the discharge diagnosis must have included diagnostic codes that most probably indicated head or spinal cord injury (Table 2-1) or diagnostic codes that suggested the possibility of nervous system injury (e.g., epilepsy). After review of each medical record, the eligible cases were followed up and interviews were arranged to assess the economic costs of head and spinal cord injury.

The major findings of the HSCI Survey are reported by Kalsbeek, McLaurin, Harris, and Miller (1980). The overall estimate of occurrence of head injury in 1974 was 422,000 cases, corresponding to an estimated incidence of 200/100,-000 population (i.e., the number of cases of head injury that were first treated as inpatients in the nation's hospitals during 1974). The incidence per 100,000 was 272 in males and 132 in females, respectively. Cases of combined head and spinal cord injury were quite rare.

The first published study of incidence applying clinical criteria of head injury severity to a defined population was reported by Annegers, Grabow, Kurland, and Laws (1980) for Olmsted County, Minnesota. The authors employed a countywide medical records linkage system, death certificates, and autopsy protocols to identify cases of head injury with evidence of "pressured brain involvement," i.e., loss of consciousness, posttraumatic amnesia, neurologic signs of brain injury, or skull fracture. The incidence per 100,000 was 274 in males and 116 in females. These figures closely approximate those obtained in the national HSCI Survey. The use of specific criteria to ascertain cases may have contributed to the relatively low incidence of head injury in the Olmsted County study, as compared to Hawthorne's findings in Scotland.

In his review of the literature concerning the epidemiology of injury to the head and spinal cord, Kraus (1980b) noted that prior to the HSCI Survey, the only published data on prevalence of head injury in the United States were from the Hospital Discharge Survey, which included a large sample of patients discharged with ICD codes 850 to 854 from hospitals located in the 50 states and the District of Columbia. The results indicated an estimated frequency of head injury of 170/100,000 population. In contrast, the HSCI Survey estimated that 926,000 head injury cases hospitalized in the years 1970 through 1974 still exhibited sequelae during 1974. The corresponding frequency (prevalence) per 100,000 population was 450, a rate considerably greater than that of the earlier Hospital Discharge Survey. The more encompassing system for eligibility of cases in the HSCI Survey could account for the higher frequency rate. A shortcoming of both studies is the exclusion of patients who died at the scene of injury or who were dead on arrival at the hospital. Moreover, the HSCI Survey yielded an undercount because patients injured before 1970 were not included, even if they were alive in 1974 and disabled by sequelae.

Data on prevalence of head injury within a community were collected by Rune (1970), who used the population of children attending primary school (ages 7 to 16) in Umea, Sweden. On the basis of parent responses to a mailed questionnaire, he found that 15% of the children had sustained a head injury that "caused the parents to worry." Nearly one-fourth of the head-injured children had been hospitalized. Cerebral "concussion" was judged to have been present in 9% of the population when a parent reported in a telephone interview that the injury produced unconsciousness, confusion persisting for at least 30 minutes, amnesia for the accident, or postconcussional symptoms. One-third of the concussed children had been hospitalized. The prevalence of head injury producing unconsciousness was 5% in the total study population. The parental report of loss of consciousness was in agreement with the medical records of those children who were hospitalized.

The third measure of morbidity employed in the National HSCI Survey was economic cost, including direct care plus indirect costs associated with the injury. On the average, the total cost of a head injury in 1974 was $2,534 ($4,114 in 1980 dollars) per injured person. The HSCI Survey disclosed that the largest average cost for head injury was for patients in the 25- to 44-year-old age group who were in the prime of their wage-earning years. Of the various etiologies of head trauma, motor vehicle accidents resulted in the most costly injuries. Kalsbeek, McLaurin, Harris, and Miller (1980) attributed this finding to more severe brain injury and possibly more frequent systemic injuries in these cases.

From the available incidence and prevalence data, closed head injury is a major public health problem in industrialized countries. The magnitude of this problem has only recently become evident through epidemiologic investigations of well-defined populations.

Cause of head injury

Field (1976) has drawn attention to the variation across studies with regard to the system for classifying cause of injury. A combination of place of occurrence (e.g., place of work) and the type of activity (e.g., industrial) is frequently used to characterize the cause of injury. Consequently, a fall may be classified as a domestic or industrial injury, depending on the study. In Table 2-2, which breaks down the cause of injury in hospital-based studies of adolescents and adults, road traffic accidents account for about one-half of all closed head injury. This finding has been confirmed by Annegers, Grabow, Kurland, and Laws (1980), Hawthorne (1978), and the National Head and Spinal Cord Injury Survey (Kalsbeek et al., 1980). In the latter study, motor vehicle accidents accounted for 70% of the head injuries that resulted in coma, but were less likely to produce an intracranial hematoma than were falls or other causes of head trauma.

Table 2-2. Cause of injury (adults)[*]

Author and country	Population	Age range and number	Road traffic accident (%)	Domestic or falls (%)	Industrial (%)	Assault (%)	Sport (%)	Other (%)
Rowbotham (1954) England	Newcastle General Hospital admissions	13 years and over (n 1000)	44	8 (domestic)	31	3	3	11
Klonoff & Thompson (1969) Canada	Visits to Emergency Department	16 years and over (n 351)	44	20 (falls)	10	13	5	8
	Admissions to neurosurgical ward (22% transferred cases)	16 years and over (n 279)	53	23 (falls)	11	4	3	6
Kerr et al. (1971) England	Newcastle General Hospital Admissions (20% transferred)	15 years and over (n 474)	48	16 (domestic)	14	13	3	6
Annegers et al. (1980) United States	Mayo Clinic countywide medical records linkage system, including death certificates (1935–74)	No age restrictions (n 3, 337)	47	29	4	4	9	7

[*]From Field, J.H. (1976). *Epidemiology of Head Injuries in England and Wales.* Department of Health and Social Security, London, and Annegers, J.F. et al. (1980). The incidence, causes and secular trends of head trauma in Olmsted County, Minnesota, 1935–74. *Neurology 30:*912–919. Reproduced with permission of the authors and publishers.

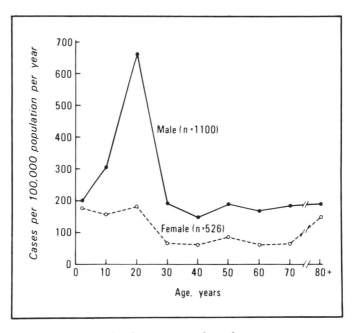

Fig. 2-1. Incidence rates of head trauma in Olmsted County, Minnesota, 1965–74. [From Annegers, J.F. et al. (1980). The incidence, causes, and secular trends of head trauma in Olmsted County, Minnesota, 1935–1974. *Neurology, 30*:912–919. Reproduced with permission of the authors and publisher.]

Age is related to cause of injury. As noted in Chapter 10, children are disproportionately injured in pedestrian–car accidents, whereas young adults and late adolescents are more often injured as occupants of motor vehicles. Falls contribute substantially to head injury in young children and in older persons. The relatively high frequency of industrial injuries in the study by Rowbotham et al., (1954) may reflect the inclusion of falls in that category. Assault producing head injury in children is frequently associated with battering by a parent.

Age

A high incidence of closed head injury in adolescents and young adults has been consistently reported (cf. Fields, 1976; Kraus, 1980b). Figure 2-1, which shows the age- and sex-specific incidence rates for head injury in Olmsted County, Minnesota, indicates a steep rise at ages 15 to 24, followed by a progressive decline until a secondary peak occurs after age 70. Head-injury admissions in children reach a peak at ages 4 to 8 (cf. Craft, 1972; Rowbotham et al., 1954).

Sex

Males consistently predominate in hospital admissions and deaths due to head
injury (Figure 2-1); the ratio of male to female hospital admissions is about 4:1,
declining to about 2:1 in patients over 70 (Fields, 1976; Kerr et al., 1971; Kraus,
1980b; Rowbotham et al., 1954). The male incidence rate rises to a peak in the
15 to 24 age range, whereas the female rate of incidence at this age is similar
to that found in the youngest age group (0 to 4). As noted in the chapter on
pediatric head injury, the male–female disparity is smaller in toddlers and pre-
school children, as compared to later childhood and adolescence.

Social class

British studies at the beginning of the past decade yielded inconsistent findings
regarding the distribution of social class in hospital admissions for head injury.
Although Steadman and Graham (1970) found little evidence for a relationship
between social class and hospital admission for head injury in Cardiff, this association was clearly demonstrated by Kerr et al. (1971) in their study of consecutive head injury admissions at the Newcastle General Hospital. Table 2-3 summarizes their findings which implicate an association between a low
socioeconomic level (their class V) and a high frequency of head injury. There
is also a trend toward an association between socioeconomic level and cause of
injury. Assault is more common in class V patients, whereas sports-related injuries figure more prominently in the upper income groups.

   This pattern of findings is in close agreement with the results of an Australian
study that was also based on consecutive head-injury admissions over a 6-year
period (Selecki, Hoy, and Ness, 1968). In a series of 910 patients, the authors
found that the occupational incidence of head injury admissions [(percentage
of total head injury admissions/percentage in population of occupational group)
× 100] was about 50% above expectation for laborers and craftsmen and about
50% below expectation for business and clerical workers and housewives. Data
from admissions for head injury in Oxford have disclosed that the overrepre-
sentation of the lower socioeconomic groups is highest in the 20- to 64-year-old
age range, particularly in patients who are 35 to 55 years old (Field, 1976).

   Although socioeconomic levels may be less strongly related to head injury in
patients at either extreme in age, Klonoff (1971) found evidence for this relationship in children. In a study of children brought to the emergency room of
the Vancouver General Hospital, he reported a disproportionately high involvement of children who lived in more congested residential areas, who had fathers
of lower occupational status, and who came from maritally unstable families.

Table 2-3. Cause of head injury in relation to social class[*]

Class[**]	Road		Domestic		Assault		Industrial		Sport		Other		Total		General population
	n	%	n	%	n	%	n	%	n	%	n	%	n	%	%
I and II	17	9.4	6	11.3	2	3.8	3	4.5	4	33.3	4	18.2	6	9.3	12.3
III	88	48.6	21	39.6	15	28.8	26	39.4	7	58.3	10	45.5	167	43.3	52.3
IV	45	24.9	9	17.0	10	19.2	28	42.4	1	8.3	5	22.7	98	25.4	21.6
V	31	17.1	17	32.1	25	48.1	9	13.6	0	—	3	13.6	85	22.0	13.8
Total	181		53		52		66		12		22		386		

[*]From Kerr, T.A., Kay, D.W., and Lassman, L.P. (1971). Characteristics of patients, type of accident, and mortality in a consecutive series of head injuries admitted to a neurosurgical unit. *Br. J. Prev. Soc. Med.* 25:179–185. Reproduced with permission of the authors and publisher.

[**]I and II denote upper social class, IV and V denote lower social class.

Risk factors

With respect to predisposing causes for injury, the use of alcohol shortly before injury is the most firmly established finding (Field, 1976; Kerr et al., 1971). Consumption of alcohol has been implicated in 29% of head injuries in males who are 15 or older and 10% of head injuries in females (Field, 1976). Depending on the study, chronic alcoholics constitute as many as one-fourth to one-half the injuries rated as being severe (Field, 1976). Alcohol also contributes immensely to closed head injuries in motor vehicle accidents and to head injuries resulting from domestic accidents and assaults (Field, 1976; Kerr et al., 1971).

Marital status was investigated by Kerr, Kay, and Lassman (1971), who found that there was a more than fourfold increase in the number of head-injured divorced persons from the number expected given their representation in the general population. This finding is compatible with the view that psychological factors contribute to the causation of accidents producing injury.

Preexisting psychiatric disorder has been cited as a factor contributing to head injury and to posttraumatic behavioral disturbance (Jennett, 1972). Although the authors of studies based on consecutive head-injury admissions have identified only a small proportion of patients with previous psychiatric conditions (cf. Kerr et al., 1971), these investigators generally have not considered the population base rate for specific psychiatric disorder nor have they applied uniform criteria and methods of examination to obtain a detailed social and psychiatric history in these patients. Contrary to the possibility of a predisposition to head injury in children, Klonoff (1971) reported that structured interviews with the parents of pediatric closed head injury patients disclosed no excess of previous head injuries, antecedent developmental anomalies, hyperactivity, mental deficiency, or emotional disturbance as compared to a control group of children matched on age, sex, grade in school, intelligence, and geographic locale. Our own experience has been that about 20% of adult hospital admissions for head injury are unsuitable for investigation of brain-behavior correlations during recovery because of previous conditions including psychiatric disorder, alcohol/drug abuse, and mental subnormality, all of which are likely to complicate their recovery and obscure the neurologic effects of injury on outcome.

Are persons who have sustained a head injury at greater risk of incurring a second injury? Annegers, Grabow, Kurland, and Laws (1980) investigated this question by comparing the incidence of subsequent head trauma after an initial head injury to the expected incidence rate for the patient's age, sex, and decade of the study, which included records from 1935–1974. They found that, after a head injury, the incidence rate is three times higher than before and that, after a second head injury, the rate increases to eight times that of the general population. The authors postulated that a behavioral pattern, in which alcohol abuse is prominent, may contribute to repeated head injury, particularly in adults.

Changes in frequency of head injury over time

Figure 2-2A shows that there was a rise of more than 40% in hospital admissions for head injury in England and Wales between 1963 and 1972. This increase primarily reflects stays of one day or less for mild injuries. Correspondingly, Figure 2-2B depicts a decline in deaths after a peak in 1964–1966. These contrasting trends have led to the inference that the number of young patients surviving head injury with residual brain damage has been increasing without, however, a proportionate expansion of rehabilitation facilities (Jennett, 1976a; London, 1967). In their study of head injury in Olmsted County, Minnesota, Annegers et al. (1980) found that the increased incidence since 1960 was primarily in the 15 to 24 age group. Further incidence studies that characterize severity of injury and outcome are necessary to determine the pattern over time of the number of brain-damaged survivors.

Seasonal and temporal variation

Head injury reaches a peak frequency in the spring in England, although the seasonal variation appeared to be of less importance than the time of day (Field, 1976). Children are more likely to suffer head injuries during the period from the end of school classes to early evening. Head injury in adults occurs most frequently from 10:00 P.M. to 4:00 A.M., particularly in alcohol-related cases.

Summary

British and American studies have shown that hospital admissions for head injury have steadily increased during the past two decades, while the number of deaths has remained constant. Although these trends suggest a rise in the number of young patients surviving head injury with varying degrees of brain damage, this hypothesis awaits confirmation by community studies of incidence

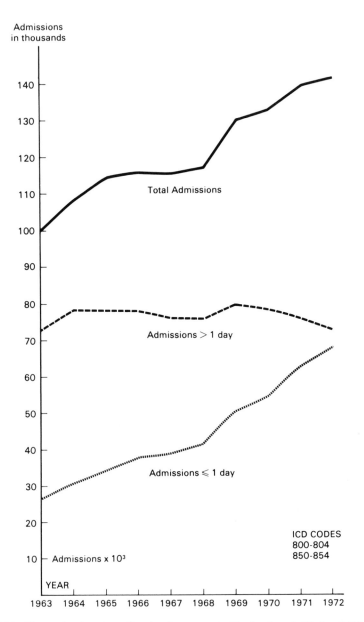

Fig. 2-2A. Hospital admissions for head injury in England and Wales, 1963–72. [Reproduced with permission of the author and the Department of Health and Social Security (UK), which commissioned this work. These items are subject to Crown Copyright and may not be reproduced without permission.)

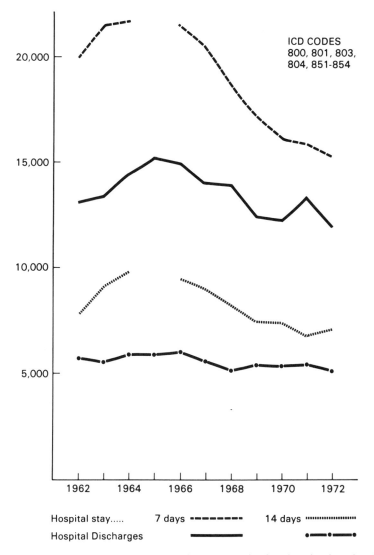

Fig. 2-2B. Deaths and discharges from head injury (England and Wales) based on hospital admissions over the same time period. [Reproduced with permission of the author and the Department of Health and Social Security (UK), which commissioned this work. These items are subject to Crown Copyright and may not be reproduced without permission.)

that include assessment of the severity of injury. Factors positively related to head injury include a history of a previous head injury, age between 15 and 30 years, male predominance, lower socioeconomic level, alcohol abuse, and divorce. The frequency of head injury also varies with the time of day and the season. Epidemiologic studies suggest that socioeconomic factors and behavior patterns may predispose toward head injury.

3. Outcome and social recovery

"Outcome" is the global term used to indicate the adequacy with which a patient's life-style is resumed, including the efficiency with which he performs the activities of daily life. Langfitt (1978) has outlined some of the reasons for measuring the outcome of closed head injury. These include providing sound information to assist clinicians in providing prognostic information to patients and their families, to assess quantitatively the effectiveness of different treatments in promoting recovery, and to document the significance of head injury as a public health problem. Langfitt also pointed out that research on outcome can provide precise information on the morbidity of closed head injury, including the costs to the individual, the family, and society. Studies of outcome also yield information required for the planning of rehabilitation facilities and the allocation of resources (Jennett, 1976a).

Mortality

Langfitt (1978) also has reviewed the reports of outcome after closed head injury that were published during the early decades of this century and concluded that, during the first quarter of the century, the mortality after severe closed head injury was 60 to 70%. Cooperative studies have analyzed the proportion of patients surviving such injury in relation to the initial impairment of consciousness, using the Glasgow Coma Scale and other indicants of severity of injury (Becker et al., 1977; Clifton et al., 1980; Jennett et al., 1976, 1977). These investigations have also considered the effects of systemic injury, as well as such individual differences as age and preinjury intelligence. In the largest series, Jennett and his coworkers (1977) selected 700 patients from the consecutive admissions for closed head injury at centers in Glasgow, the Netherlands (Groningen, Rotterdam), and Los Angeles. The criterion for admission to this international data bank was a Coma Scale score of 7 or less for a period of at least six hours, beginning with the initial evaluation in the emergency room. This criterion implied that there was no eye opening, an inability to utter recognizable words, and a failure to follow commands. There was variation across the four centers in the interval between the time of injury and admission to a neurosurgical service. Patients in Glasgow were referred from primary care centers because of surgical lesions or neurologic deterioration, whereas patients generally were admitted directly to the other hospitals participating in the study. The data in Table 3-1, however, show a relatively uniform mortality of approximately 50% at each center.

Subsequent investigations of outcome after severe closed head injury have indicated that rapid evacuation to a neurosurgical center, with prompt assessment by CT scanning and initiation of definitive treatment, can prevent or even reverse secondary brain injury (Becker et al., 1977; Bowers and Marshall, 1980; Clifton et al., 1980; Marshall et al., 1979a,b; Miller et al., 1981). Studies from the Medical College of Virginia (Becker et al., 1977; Miller et al., 1981) and the University of California, San Diego (Marshall et al., 1979a,b) have reported a lower mortality (Table 3-1), as compared to the findings in the three-country study of Jennett and colleagues. The authors of the Virginia and San Diego studies attributed the apparent reduction in mortality to early treatment to control raised intracranial pressure and to rapid surgical removal of hematomas and pulped brain acting as mass lesions. Clifton et al. (1980) also reported a mortality of about 30% using a treatment protocol simiar to that employed in the Richmond and San Diego studies. In contrast to previous investigations, three-fourths of the patients in Clifton's study were evacuated by a helicopter ambulance, which was staffed by a trauma team including a surgery resident and a nurse. The differences in mortality may also reflect heterogeneity in the head injuries despite efforts (cf. Miller et al., 1981) to select patients according to the criteria developed by Jennett and his colleagues. Langfitt (1981) has proposed a "holistic" classification of head injury that would encompass the Glasgow Coma Scale, the pathology indicated by CT, and the patient's age.

From these studies, we may conclude that a patient who sustains a head injury of sufficient severity to be rated below 8 on the Glasgow Coma Scale has a 50 to 70% chance of survival with the best current therapy. Neuropathologic

Table 3-1. Comparison of outcome for severely head injured patient

	Glasgow[°] (n 428)	Netherlands[°] (n 172)	Los Angeles[°] (n 100)	Richmond[°°] (n 160)	San Diego[†] (n 200)	Richmond[‡] (n 225)
Dead	221 (52%)	89 (52%)	49 (49%)	48 (30%)	72 (36%)	76 (34%)
Vegetative state	8 (2%)	1 (1%)	5 (5%)	4 (2%)	8 (4%)	7 (3%)
Severe disability	34 (8%)	9 (5%)	18 (18%)	12 (8%)	16 (8%)	16 (7%)
Moderate disability	71 (17%)	26 (15%)	14 (14%)	39 (24%)	20 (10%)	25 (11%)
Good recovery	94 (22%)	47 (27%)	14 (14%)	57 (36%)	84 (42%)	101 (45%)

Note that the data from Richmond include patients who were not compatible with the international data bank (e.g., a duration of coma less than six ho urs), although all patients were incapable of obeying commands on admission.

[°]From Jennett et al. (1977). Three-country study. The Dutch centers were Groningen and Rotterdam.

[°°]From Becker et al. (1977).

[†]From Bowers and Marshall (1980). Glasgow Coma Scale score ≤7 for six hours or more.

[‡]From Miller et al. (1981).

study of primary impact versus secondary damage to the brain in patients dying after head injury suggests that the incidence of irreversible brain damage at the time of impact in motor vehicle accidents may be about 25% and that the survival may never exceed 75% for injuries occurring in vehicular accidents that produce a score of 7 or less (Clifton et al., 1980).

The question of prediction of outcome based on neurologic indicants of the severity of injury is considered in detail by Jennett and Teasdale (1981). Several investigators have found that the Glasgow Coma Scale provides a more confident prognosis when serial scores, rather than only the initial score at the time of admission, are considered (Braakman et al., 1980; Clifton et al., 1980; Jennett et al., 1976). In these and other studies, the presence of such neurologic indicants as nonreactive pupils and oculovestibular deficit has been related to increased mortality (Becker et al., 1977; Jennett et al., 1976). Becker et al. reported that patients with mass lesions generally had a poorer prognosis than patients with diffuse closed head injuries. Jennett and Teasdale (1981) reviewed the effects of age on outcome and found that within a series of closed head injury patients, in which the total Glasgow Coma Scale score was below 8 for a period of six hours or more, the probability of death increased exponentially as a function of age at the time of injury. Other findings have suggested that patients above 50 years old are more likely to have acute subdural hematoma. Alcoholism also more frequently complicates the injuries of older patients.

Morbidity

Outcome studies of severe closed head injury at different centers have characterized the quality of recovery in global terms on the basis of social functioning, vocational adjustment, and physical disability.

Carlsson, Von Essen, and Lofgren (1968) proposed the criterion of "mental restitution," which they defined as the "mental capacity of these patients (diffuse CHI) to resume their former work or active rehabilitation in the presence of residual paresis or other disablements." This broad, dichotomous measure of outcome includes both patients who have fully recovered and cases with residual disability who undergo rehabilitation. Presumably, "unrestituted" cases included those who were severely disabled or vegetative. Of 320 closed head injury patients who survived a period of coma of at least 12 hours, the authors judged that 83% were "mentally reconstituted." They also found that the time required to achieve this criterion of recovery was directly related to the duration of coma.

Standardization in the assessment of global outcome has been facilitated by the development of the Glasgow Outcome Scale to categorize closed head injury patients on the basis of their physical and economic dependence and social reintegration (Jennett and Bond, 1975). This scale describes four levels of recovery: persistent vegetative state (PVS); severe disability (SD); moderate disability (MD); and good recovery (GR). Each category of outcome is a composite of cognitive, physical, and social functioning. Although the persistent vegetative state and good recovery ratings of outcome are fairly unequivocal, designation of outcome within the middle range of recovery is more difficult. Some authors have presented their outcome results by merging the categories of good recovery and moderate disability (cf. Langfitt, 1978; Marshall et al., 1979 a,b). However, Levin, Grossman, Rose, and Teasdale (1979) found that the moderate disability category encompasses a wide range of neuropsychological functioning and social adjustment. Therefore, they use the followup neurologic examination, interviews with the patient and family, and the results of neuropsychological testing to characterize outcome within the moderate and severe disability grades.

Persistent vegetative state

Jennett and Plum (1972) proposed that the term persistent vegetative state be used to describe patients who remain speechless and devoid of meaningful contact with other persons. Such patients frequently open their eyes and exhibit sleep-waking cycles. Clinical experience indicates that some cases classified as in a persistent vegetative state at three to six months may improve subsequently and progress to the severe disability category.

Widespread injury to the cerebral white matter and lesions of the brain stem have been implicated in persistent vegetative states (Adams et al., 1977; Strich, 1970). In view of the clear definition of the state offered by Jennett and Plum, the wide disparities in the percentages of these patients across outcome studies (Table 3-1) is unexpected. In Table 3-1, the discrepancy in frequency of persistent vegetative states is as great as fourfold. Variation in the delay preceding definitive treatment, in the adequacy of treatment, or in the age of patients may be contributory. An otherwise fatal course may result in a vegetative outcome depending upon the mode of emergency evacuation and treatment protocol.

In an epidemiologic study involving 269 hospitals in Japan, Higashi et al. (1977) applied specific criteria to ascertain the overall incidence of the persistent vegetative state, as (1) defective verbal and behavioral communication; (2) loss of expression of intention; (3) absence (or at least reduction) of emotional

expression; (4) urinary and fecal incontinence; (5) complete loss of self-support-
ability; (6) continuation of the above conditions for more than three months.
Accordingly, they identified 100 patients, including 38 closed head injury cases,
and estimated the population incidence to be 0.0025%. In contrast to persistent
vegetative state from other causes, the mean survival time of closed head injury
patients was 33 months (SD = 26); 45% of these patients were still alive at the
end of the 3-year followup interval. The followup data supported Jennett and
Plum's designation of this condition as "persistent." Only three patients became
communicative over the course of the study. It should be noted, however, that
patients frequently pass through a phase of vegetative state during the course
of recovery from severe closed head injuries.

Severe disability

Jennett and Bond described patients who were severely disabled as "dependent
for daily support by reason of mental or physical disability, usually a combination of both." Although severely disabled patients are usually institutional-
ized, the authors acknowledged that exceptional family support may enable
some patients to reside at home. Although the patients may show neurologic
deficits as a result of their head injury, these deficits generally improve in the
first year after injury, although their postinjury intellectual and memory deficits
and behavioral disturbance persist. The net result is severe functional disability.
In contrast to persistent vegetative state patients, the severely disabled patient
is capable of some communication (though aphasia may be present), ambulation, and some degree of self-care. Table 3-2 depicts the proportion of each

Table 3-2. Comparison of outcome in survivors of severe head injury at different
centers[°]

Series	No. of cases	Good recovery		Moderate disability		Severe disability		Persistent vegetative state	
		n	%	n	%	n	%	n	%
Galveston	27	10	37	12	44	5	19	0	0
Glasgow	207	94	45	71	34	34	16	8	5
Los Angeles	51	14	28	14	28	18	35	5	9
Netherlands[°°]	83	47	57	26	31	9	11	1	1
Richmond	112	57	51	39	35	12	10	4	4
San Diego	128	84	66	20	16	16	12	8	6

[°] Patients who died are excluded.
[°°] Groningen, Rotterdam

outcome category among survivors of severe closed head injury in various series. It is clear that the frequency of severe disability varied considerably in the different series of patients. For example, severe disability was more than three times as common among patients treated in Los Angeles than among those treated in the Netherlands.

Moderate disability

This outcome is used to designate patients who can utilize public transportation and can work in a sheltered environment, i.e., those who are independent in daily activities. Residual motor and neuropsychological deficits are compatible with moderate disability, as are major personality changes and family disruption. Rating of disability, however, is occasionally complicated by the presence of severe focal deficits that impair functioning, despite adequate recovery in other areas. For example, two closed head injury patients hospitalized in Galveston, who had sustained massive right hemisphere hematomas, showed residual neglect of the left visual field that prevented them from compensating for visual field defects. Consequently, they were unable to attend to household responsibilities and could not use public transportation. Despite satisfactory recovery of verbal ability, both patients were severely disabled during the first year of their recovery.

Good recovery

Jennett and Bond did not use resumption of work as a criterion of good recovery because employment may depend upon local economic conditions and other extrinsic factors, such as variation in disability benefits and type of work. Conversely, patients may return to work in a family business or in a noncompetitive setting despite considerable neuropsychological impairment.

The severity of injury, as measured by coma score or coma duration, is related to subsequent employment. Of 27 young adult patients with initial Glasgow Coma scores below 8, Levin, Grossman, Rose, and Teasdale (1979) found that only 12 (44%) were employed at the time of followup (an average of one year after injury). Nine of these patients (33%) were categorized as having made a good recovery. Only one of 12 moderately disabled patients was fully employed and two were working part time. Consistent with these results, Oddy, Humphrey, and Uttley (1978) reported that employment 6 months after a closed head injury was closely associated with the duration of posttraumatic amnesia. Similarly, Gilchrist and Wilkinson (1979) found that duration of unconsciousness, but not focal neurologic deficit, was significantly related to the likelihood of eventually returning to work. In a similar followup study of 50 closed head injury patients who had been "deeply unconscious" for at least 24 hours, Thomsen (1974) found that only four cases (8%) had resumed their preinjury work 30 months after injury, whereas 36 (72%) were not engaged in any vocational activity. Residual disability at the time of followup was attributable to motor handicap in only 10 patients (20%). More encouraging results were reported by Gilchrist and Wilkinson (1979) who found that of 70 closed head injury patients under 40 years of age at the time of injury, 39% were working at the time of a followup (nine months to 15 years after injury). The patients studied by Gilchrist and Wilkinson were drawn from rehabilitation units in London, which may have excluded cases with other debilitating conditions such as alcoholism. Return to work was investigated by Denny-Brown (1945) in 200 nearly consecutive closed head injury admissions to the Boston City Hospital who were followed for at least six months. Of this series, 170 had varying degrees of deficit attributable to head injury rather than extracranial complications or preexisting conditions. Ninety-two percent of these patients returned to work by six months after injury. In contrast to the aforementioned studies, only four patients (2%) were unconscious for periods longer than 24 hours. Denny-Brown found that prolonged temporal disorientation and acute neurologic deficit were related to subsequent unemployment as was the development of anxiety-related symptoms, which frequently constituted a posttraumatic syndrome. From the above, it would appear that the resumption of work is a useful, if not entirely satisfactory criterion of quality of recovery as related to severity of initial injury.

Striking variation in the proportion of patients achieving a good recovery is depicted in Table 3-2. In the San Diego series, the relative frequency of a good recovery was more than twice that of the Los Angeles study. In a long-term outcome study (Levin et al., 1979), which was confined to patients without previous neuropsychiatric disorder, the relative frequency of good recovery in young adults was closer to that found in the Los Angeles study. Neuropsychological correlates of good recovery in this study included an IQ within the average range, resolution of aphasic defect, and no more than mild behavioral disturbances. Acute neurologic findings in patients who eventually attained a good recovery were compared to those cases who were unable to fully resume their previous responsibilities. In contrast to patients who became functionally disabled, no patient with a good recovery initially exhibited bilaterally nonreactive pupils or oculovestibular disturbance. Although hemiparesis and coma duration exceeding one day were less common in patients who achieved a good recovery, there was marked individual variation. Good recovery (63%) among the 100 consecutive patients described by Marshall, Smith, and Shapiro (1979a,b), however, was found in patients who initially had nonreactive pupils or oculovestibular deficit. Raised intracranial pressure more clearly differentiated the disabled from the fully recovered patients than did any other indicant of initial injury severity.

Outcome data based largely on assessment of activities of daily living lack sufficient detail to characterize residual social functioning, family relationships, and recreational activities. Structured interviews (see Appendix A) have disclosed that long-term recovery from severe closed head injury frequently results in diminution of social contacts and withdrawal to isolated activities. Disruption of marriage is a common sequel of severe closed head injury. Clinical experience suggests that eventual divorce of the injured partner by the spouse is almost the rule if a moderate or severe disability is the long-term outcome of injury. A pattern of disturbed social functioning and reduced leisure activities was confirmed by Oddy, Humphrey, and Uttley (1978) and Oddy and Humphrey (1980), who obtained ratings on the Katz Social Adjustment Scale from relatives. In the 1979 study, followup data at six months postinjury showed that patients with a posttraumatic amnesia duration exceeding seven days had a decline in the number of close friends, a decrease in the frequency of social outings, and a reciprocal rise in loneliness. Oddy and Humphrey (1980) found that reduced social and leisure activities persisted at two years postinjury, although 90% of the patients with severe closed head injuries had returned to work. Loss of contact with friends was also described by Thomsen (1974). Gronwall has postulated that a residual impairment in capacity for information processing, particularly in situations with multiple speakers and conversations, might contribute to the social retreat in many patients. Diminished insight regarding limitations after severe closed head injury has been described by several authors (Gronwall, 1976b; Jennett, 1976b; Levin and Grossman, 1978). Chronically disabled patients sometimes show marked lack of concern and they may display a euphoric or fatuous mood.

Summary

Investigations of outcome after closed head injury have focused primarily on survival and adequacy of social and vocational functioning. In view of the outcome studies reported during the past decades, it appears that optimal emergency evacuation and neurosurgical treatment may reduce the mortality from severe closed head injury to 25 to 30% (Clifton et al., 1981). Serial Glasgow

Coma scores, pupillary findings, and oculovestibular testing have been the best neurologic predictors of survival. Of the demographic variables, age has been shown to have the greatest prognostic significance. Estimates of the frequency of good recovery (i.e., resumption of preinjury life-style) have varied across studies. A review of the literature and our own experience suggest that one-fourth to one-third of patients admitted with severe closed head injuries (or about one-third to one-half of the survivors) can achieve a good recovery with optimal treatment.

4. Anterograde and retrograde amnesia

Anterograde amnesia, i.e., loss of memory for events after trauma or disease onset, is probably the most consistent clinical feature of closed head injury. Symonds (1962) compared anterograde amnesia after head injury to the pervasive memory disorder caused by bilateral temporal lobectomy and herpes simplex encephalitis involving the temporal lobes. He postulated that amnesia associated with closed head injury is produced by axonal shearing in the anterior temporal region. Distortion and stretching of nerve fibers, which may transiently arrest function without causing degeneration, may account for the eventual resolution of the amnesia. Jennett (1969) drew attention to the vulnerability of the temporal lobes to surface contusions, intracerebral hematoma, tentorial herniation, and hypoxia.

Posttraumatic amnesia and its measurement

Russell (1932) proposed that the criterion of "the duration of loss of full consciousness" be utilized to characterize the severity of closed head injury. In a series of 200 patients, he estimated this duration on the basis of retrospective report by the patient of when he "woke up." The interval from the time of injury to the patient's remembrance of waking up was designated as the duration of disturbed consciousness. Russell and Nathan (1946) then introduced the term posttraumatic amnesia for the phenomenon. At the same time, they modified the original criterion to include the patient's capacity to become "suffi-

74 CLOSED HEAD INJURY

EARLY STAGES OF RECOVERY FROM CLOSED HEAD INJURY

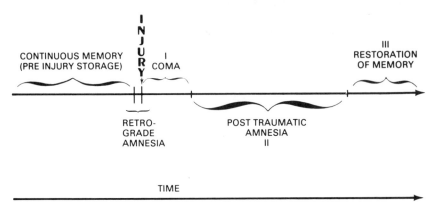

Fig. 4-1. Sequence of acute alterations in memory after closed head injury. The periods of coma (I) and posttraumatic amnesia (II) have been traditionally combined to yield a total interval of impaired consciousness that extends until continuous memory for ongoing events (III) is restored.

ciently aware of his surroundings to commit them to memory." As in Russell's 1932 study, the duration of posttraumatic amnesia was, in fact, a combination of the periods of coma and of the confusional phase of recovery. Retrospective reports obtained after the amnesic period were used to estimate the duration of the amnesia. The definition of posttraumatic amnesia duration was further refined by Russell and Smith (1961) as "the length of the interval during which current events have not been stored." According to this definition, posttraumatic amnesia following coma (Figure 4-1) is used synonymously with anterograde amnesia. Although we use these terms interchangeably to refer to the period of gross confusion and amnesia for ongoing events after the patient emerges from coma, it is important to recognize that Russell and his colleagues included both the length of coma and the period of anterograde amnesia in their estimation of the total duration of posttraumatic amnesia.

Duration of posttraumatic amnesia as an index of closed head injury severity gained wide acceptance in Great Britain through the dissemination of findings by Russell and his colleagues at the Oxford Head Injury Hospital during and after World War II on patients who had been treated at the Military Hospital for Head Injuries in Oxford. These studies demonstrated that the duration of posttraumatic amnesia was fairly predictive of long-term recovery in military personnel who had sustained blunt head injury. It was found to be particularly useful in the case of patients in whom details of the initial injury were unavailable.

Careful questioning after recovery of consciousness and normal orientation was again advocated by Russell (1971) as a means of determining the beginning of continuous memory for ongoing events (Figure 4-1). The retrospective method was defended on the grounds that a recently injured patient might be aware of his surroundings, but still be unable to store ongoing events. Reports of head-injured football, baseball, and golf players carrying out sequential plays for which they were later amnesic attest to the range of complex activity observed immediately after mild closed head injury (cf. Bogen, 1980; Yarnell and Lynch, 1970). The presence of "islands of memory," i.e., memory of a postinjury event followed by a period of amnesia, was also cited by Russell as a source of measurement error if posttraumatic amnesia were measured during the early phase of recovery rather than by retrospective report. Gronwall and Wrightson (1980) recently reported that islands of memory were present in more than one-third of cases with a minor closed head injury. Russell (1932, 1935) considered posttraumatic amnesia to be primarily useful in determining severity of injury in patients without focal mass lesion. The method proved to be very valuable in the first systematic clinical studies of outcome after closed head injury, which continue to be of great significance (Russell, 1935; Russell and Nathan, 1946; Russell and Smith, 1961).

Querying the patient retrospectively, however, is open to criticism because of the inherent difficulty he may experience in differentiating information about the injury given him by family members after termination of posttraumatic amnesia from information obtained at an earlier point in recovery. Russell and his associates defined duration of the amnesia without providing uniform criteria of proven reliability for its measurement. As we have seen, assessment of coma can be unreliable in the absence of strict criteria (Teasdale et al., 1978). In view of the reduction in measurement error found by Teasdale et al. for the Glasgow Coma Scale, as compared to unstructured clinical assessment, it is reasonable to suggest that quantitative assessment of posttraumatic amnesia would be more reliable than unstructured clinical judgment. Gronwall and Wrightson (1980) have recently shown discrepancies between retrospective estimates of duration of amnesia by patients who recovered from mild closed head injury and direct measurement of amnesia by serial interviews while they were in the hospital.

Posttraumatic amnesia and coma

In Russell's method of assessing the severity of brain injury by estimating the duration of disturbed consciousness, there was no partitioning of the phases of coma and of subsequent confusion in measuring the duration of posttraumatic amnesia (cf. Figure 4-1). Accordingly, an amnesia of 10 days, consisting of two days of coma and eight days of confusion/disorientation, presumably would be considered to be functionally equivalent to a posttraumatic amnesia of equal total duration, in which four days of coma were followed by six days of confusion. This undifferentiated approach inevitably raises the question of the relationship between the duration of coma as defined by the Glasgow Coma Scale (or some other criterion) and the period of residual anterograde amnesia. Given serial ratings on the Glasgow Coma Scale, is it possible to predict the subsequent interval of disorientation and confusion?

Von Wowern (1966) compared estimates of posttraumatic amnesia based on retrospective interviews with the duration of coma as determined from hospital records. There was a lack of correspondence between the duration of coma and amnesia, particularly in patients over 50 years old. However, one must be cautious in drawing conclusions from Von Wowern's study, since both variables were retrospective in nature and the definition of coma was not precise. Clinical experience indicates that many closed head injury patients have protracted periods of disorientation and confusion despite very brief durations of coma. Indeed, discrepancies between the duration of coma and the period of subsequent confusion were reported by Ruesch and Moore as early as 1943.

A wide disparity between the duration of coma and the period of anterograde amnesia is exemplified in the case of a 65-year-old woman who was rendered unconscious for only a few minutes after she was struck on the head by an assailant on 9 January 1981. Examination in the emergency room 20 minutes after injury disclosed spontaneous eye opening, ability to obey commands, and confused, but coherent speech (Glasgow Coma Scale score of 14). A CT scan on the day of injury visualized hemorrhagic contusions in the left temporal and right frontal areas without evidence of mass effect. Although there were no signs of neurologic deterioration or clinically apparent aphasia, the patient remained disoriented and confused for 12 days. Neuropsychological assessment on 21 January disclosed her orientation to be at the lower limit of normal, despite repeated prompting by the nursing staff during her hospital stay. She could not recall visiting the neuropsychology laboratory for the morning session when she returned after lunch to complete the assessment. She misestimated her hospital stay as one month in duration and could not describe current events (e.g., the release of the American hostages in Iran), although she had frequently viewed news programs on television. In summary, the duration of this patient's disorientation and confusion was prolonged far beyond her transient period of unconsciousness. It is conceivable that her age contributed to this disparity.

The measurement of posttraumatic amnesia maintains its usefulness as an index of the severity of injury, particularly since increasing use of intubation and the administration of barbiturates may alter the significance of ratings on coma scales.

Posttraumatic amnesia and disorientation

Moore and Ruesch (1944) studied recovery of orientation to time, place, and context in 39 patients hospitalized after closed head injuries. Each day they presented a standard series of questions to test orientation and found that readiness for detailed psychological testing coincided with the recovery of orientation. Although Moore and Ruesch did not report later retrospective estimates of posttraumatic amnesia by their patients, they suggested that the resolution of amnesia paralleled that of disorientation, concluding that "the duration of confusion (disorientation) is the best criterion for evaluation of the severity of damage to mental function."

The possibility that disorientation and anterograde amnesia are manifestations of a common underlying deficit during the early stage of recovery has not received consistent support. Wowern found that the interval of posttraumatic amnesia estimated from retrospective report by patients long after injury corresponded closely to the note in the hospital chart indicating that the patient was "alert and oriented." As noted by Schacter and Crovitz (1977), replication of Wowern's study by direct daily monitoring of orientation is needed to draw firm conclusions. Correspondence between duration of anterograde amnesia and disorientation was reported in only one-half the patients studied by Sisler and Penner (1975), who focused on very mild injuries treated in the emergency room.

In a study of patients with closed head injury of varying severity, Artiola i Fortuny, and her coworkers (1980) used the consistent retention of simple items over a 24-hour interval to define the termination of posttraumatic amnesia. It was found that this measure of amnesia yielded durations that were similar to the estimates made by neurosurgeons who had interviewed the patients on the ward. Gronwall and Wrightson (1980) measured posttraumatic amnesia in the emergency room after minor closed head injury by serially questioning the patients about postinjury events. Their results indicated that the return of continuous memory for ongoing events and normal orientation (assessed by a brief test) were not coincident. It will be necessary to study a more heterogeneous series of closed head injury patients to determine which measure is more useful to characterize the initial period of disorientation and anterograde amnesia.

Duration of posttraumatic amnesia

In a monograph summarizing his experience with closed head injuries in British servicemen evacuated to Oxford, Russell (1971) presented an overall distribution of posttraumatic amnesia durations (Table 4-1). He divided the cases into four subgroups according to the delay between the time of injury and admission to the Military Hospital for Head Injuries. The groups with longer delays (particularly Group D) generally had more severe injuries than those transferred earlier. From the data in Table 4-1, Russell inferred that a posttraumatic amnesia exceeding seven days is indicative of severe generalized injury, whereas one of less than one hour suggests mild injury.

Schacter and Crovitz (1977) have cautioned that the clinical significance of posttraumatic amnesia duration may vary with both the method of measurement and the selection of patients. In agreement with the widely held view that closed head injuries have more devastating effects on older individuals, Russell

Table 4-1. Comparisons of percent of invalidism with increasing posttraumatic amnesia (PTA) intervals in the four groups of British military closed head injury patients° transferred to the Oxford Hospital

	Group	Total No.	Total %	Nil No.	Nil %	<1 hr No.	<1 hr %	1–24 hr No.	1–24 hr %	1–7 days No.	1–7 days %	>7 days No.	>7 days %
PTA	A	186	—	23	12	75	40	51	27	13	7	24	13
	B	168	—	14	8	44	26	37	22	39	23	34	20
	C	661	—	59	9	117	8	224	34	156	24	105	16
	D	309	—	19	6	36	11	67	22	99	31	88	29
Invalided	A		11		0		1		9		15		54
	B		27		14		20		24		23		47
	C		58		44		53		58		60		67
	D		44		42		44		33		42		56

From Russell, W.R. (1971). *The Traumatic Amnesias*, Oxford University Press. Reproduced with permission of the publisher.

°Group A, admission to Oxford Hospital within three days of injury
 Group B, admission to Oxford Hospital within three weeks of injury
 Group C, admission after 3 weeks because of difficulties in rehabilitation or treatment
 Group D, severe injuries admitted after three weeks to Oxford

and Smith (1961) found that the distribution of posttraumatic amnesia in older patients was skewed towards prolonged intervals.

Behavioral manifestations of posttraumatic amnesia

Patients recovering from closed head injuries (n 86) or penetrating gunshot wounds (n 9), who had been comatose for at least eight hours, were serially interviewed by Weinstein and Lyerly (1968) in order to study anomalous cognitive processes during the subacute phase of recovery. Confabulation (invention of a story about a past event or a gross distortion of an actual occurrence) was exhibited by 60% of the patients; themes about other people and personal violence predominated. Demographic variables such as age and education were not related to the presence of confabulation nor was the severity of injury (although the latter was not clearly defined). In most cases, confabulation was elicited by questions about the patient's disability and the circumstances surrounding admission to the hospital. Although the authors did not report concurrent measures of orientation, it is likely that this improved as the confabulation diminished.

Benson, Gardner, and Meadows (1976) have described the early recovery of two patients who had sustained severe closed head injuries that rendered them comatose and/or confused for prolonged periods. After posttraumatic amnesia had at least partially cleared (as evidenced by their ability to recall the date, the names of their doctors and the hospital, and the details of the accident reported to them), the patients consistently mislocated the hospital (reduplicative paramnesia) as a place that held significance for them earlier in their lives. From these observations it would appear important to inquire about geographic orientation and the patient's interpretation of the injury when assessing posttraumatic amnesia.

Delusional thinking and hallucinations may accompany confabulation. In such cases it is not inappropriate to describe the early period of recovery as a transient posttraumatic psychosis, as described in Chapter 9.

Retrograde amnesia

Retrograde amnesia is defined by Russell (1971) as "the interval preceding the injury, of which the patient has no recollection." As with posttraumatic amnesia, he estimated the duration of retrograde amnesia by questioning the patient after return of "full consciousness," i.e., normal orientation and restoration of continuous memory. Table 4-2 depicts the correspondence between posttrau-

Table 4-2. Duration of posttraumatic amnesia (PTA) and retrograde amnesia (RA) compared in 1,029 cases of "accidental" head injury (gunshot wounds excluded) admitted to Oxford Hospital.

Duration of RA	Duration of PTA						
	Nil	<1 hr	1–24 hr	1–7 days	>7 days	No record	Total
Nil	99	23	9	2	0	0	133
Under 30 minutes	—	178	274	174	80	1	707
Over 30 minutes	—	3	16	41	73	0	133
No record°	—	4	14	14	15	9	56
Total	99	208	313	231	168	10	1,029

From Russell, W.R. and Nathan, P.W. (1946). *Brain* 69:280–300. Reproduced with permission of the publisher.
°Retrograde amnesia duration was available for 973 patients, posttraumatic amnesia duration was available for 1,019 cases.

matic and retrograde amnesia durations in a large sample of closed head injury cases, most of whom were seen at the Military Hospital for Head Injuries in Oxford (Russell and Nathan, 1946). Retrograde amnesia lasted less than 30 minutes in over 80% of the total series and generally was brief in relation to posttraumatic amnesia; it lasted less than 30 minutes in about 50% of the patients who had posttraumatic amnesia exceeding seven days. The high frequency of retrograde amnesia of brief duration documented in Table 4-2 led Russell and Nathan to suggest that it had a clear and uniform physiologic basis. Possibly the cerebral insult disrupts consolidation of memory by blocking its transfer from the labile short-term memory to permanent storage.

In view of the relatively weak correlation between range of variation in retrograde amnesia duration and posttraumatic amnesia duration, Russell and his colleagues concluded that the former was a less accurate index of severity. However, in a subsequent study of patients with mild closed head injuries, Bromlert and Sisler (1974) interviewed patients in the emergency room who had already recovered from a brief period of coma or "circumscribed amnesia." The results showed a somewhat stronger correspondence between retrograde and posttraumatic amnesia durations. When the latter was less than one hour, the former did not exceed one minute.

Russell (1935) suggested that a residual retrograde amnesia extending for periods longer than a few weeks represented a hysterical manifestation. Against this view, Symonds (1962) described two closed head injury patients in whom retrospective interviews disclosed a retrograde amnesia duration of three months with a posttraumatic amnesia duration of four weeks in one case and a retrograde amnesia duration of one year with a posttraumatic amnesia of five weeks in the other. Symonds denied that the retrograde amnesia had a hysterical basis in these patients and he invoked more rapid forgetting of events in the remote past as an explanation (Symonds, 1966).

Shrinking retrograde amnesia

Russell (1935) described this feature of posttraumatic memory disorder in a closed head injury patient who exhibited a retrograde amnesia of nine years' duration during the transition from coma to resolution of posttraumatic amnesia. Over a period of ten weeks, he gradually recollected events in the remote past beginning with the earliest memories and finally recalled everything within a few minutes of the motorcycle accident. Russell and Nathan (1946) confirmed this pattern in other cases in which they found that in retrograde amnesia, memories were recovered in chronological order beginning with those from the distant past with later filling in of recent events. They noted that shrinkage of retrograde amnesia usually paralleled resolution of posttraumatic amnesia, although they cited exceptional cases in which gaps in the past persisted in normally oriented patients.

Shrinking retrograde amnesia was later described by Benson and Geschwind (1967) in a patient who had a right temporal subgaleal hematoma of undetermined etiology who was "stuporous but not really unconscious." During the early phase of recovery, a retrograde amnesia of two years' duration was exhibited; responses to questions concerning address, occupation, and family life corresponded to the patient's life two years prior to injury (e.g., he insisted that he was living in Washington, D.C., although he had moved to Boston two years before). After a period of three months, recall of remote information steadily improved until the patient was left with a residual gap of 24 hours prior to admission. The authors conjectured that the patient's probable alcoholic intoxication shortly before injury extended the period of permanent retrograde amnesia. They contrasted the brief residual retrograde amnesia after head injury with the permanent one in metabolic Korsakoff's disease, which may span periods as long as several decades. The shrinkage of retrograde amnesia was interpreted as evidence for gradual restoration of retrieval of memories from long-term storage; posttraumatic amnesia was interpreted as reflecting impaired consolidation of new information. Although the inability to recall salient remote information, which undoubtedly was consolidated prior to injury, constitutes strong evidence for a retrieval hypothesis of retrograde amnesia, there is no reason to doubt that impaired retrieval also contributes to deficient learning and memory after head injury. As described in Chapter 5, recent studies have suggested that the process of searching the contents of long-term storage appears to be particularly vulnerable to the effects of closed head injury. In any case, elucidation of the parallel between shrinkage of retrograde amnesia and clearing of posttraumatic amnesia deserves further study.

Measurement of retrograde amnesia and its temporal gradient

Schacter and Crovitz (1977) concluded that "the single greatest deficiency in the literature concerned with RA [retrograde amnesia] following closed head trauma is the lack of appropriate methods which permit quantitative study of the phenomenon." The retrospective interview used by Russell and his colleagues to assess retrograde amnesia was not quantitative, and the data are subject to distortion arising from the patient's incorporation of information provided by relatives into his account of events preceding the injury. Moreover, there is no standardization of the questioning or of the criteria for determining the border between continuous memory prior to injury and retrograde amnesia (Figure 4-1). Events preceding the injury are difficult to verify and are vulnerable to normal forgetting even in the absence of a head injury. Probing about events from the distant past is often confined to information that has been well rehearsed and overlearned prior to the injury (e.g., birthplace). Studies of both animals (Orbach and Fantz, 1958) and human subjects (Benton, Levin, and Van Allen, 1974) have established that overlearned material is less vulnerable to disruption by cerebral insult.

Memory for remote events has been investigated primarily in patients with severe anterograde amnesia secondary to Korsakoff's disease and those who have undergone bilateral mesial temporal lobe resection. Remote memory has also been studied in normal aging. These studies have evaluated the dictum of Ribot (1882) that the extent of memory loss for any past event is inversely related to the time since its occurrence. Anecdotal observations of closed head injury patients during the confusional stage of recovery suggest that their oldest memories are more resistant to the effects of brain trauma (Russell, 1935). The practical significance of a temporal gradient lies in the clinician's ability to estimate loss of previously acquired information, particularly with respect to the patient's occupation or curriculum in school.

Attempts to quantify and standardize assessment of remote memory have consisted mainly of recall and recognition tasks for news events and photographs of individuals who figured prominently in past decades (cf. Albert, Butters, and Levin, 1979; Warrington and Sanders, 1971). Discontinuity between preserved memory for events and for faces of public figures in the news prior to the onset of anterograde amnesia was found by Marslen-Wilson and Teuber (1975) in alcoholic Korsakoff patients and in a patient who had undergone bilateral temporal lobectomy. A temporal gradient of retrograde amnesia was confirmed by Squire and Slater (1978) by testing the recall of news events in a patient who developed an amnesic disorder after receiving a stab wound to the basal brain. No gradient was found, however, when a multiple choice test was given. Support for Ribot's postulate was provided by Albert, Butters, and Levin (1979) who reported a steep temporal gradient with preservation of the oldest memories in alcoholic patients with Korsakoff's disease independently of the method of testing (recall, recognition), format of memoranda (photographs, questions on past events), or level of difficulty (easy vs. difficult items). The finding of a temporal gradient confirmed the reports of Marslen-Wilson and Teuber (1975) and Seltzer and Benson (1974). In contrast to these results, Sanders and Warrington (1971) found that remote memory in five amnesic patients (including three Korsakoff cases) was impaired for information spanning a 50-year period without evidence of less severe disruption of older items. Studies using similar techniques have also failed to demonstrate sparing of the most remote memories in the elderly (Squire, 1974; Warrington and Sanders, 1971).

From this review of clinical and gerontologic studies of remote memory, it may be concluded that a temporal gradient in retention of past events is not universal. There is no disagreement, however, that retrograde amnesia is manifested by patients with Korsakoff's disease and by patients with surgical lesions of the mesial temporal lobes. The mechanisms underlying retrograde amnesia in Korsakoff's disease and bilateral temporal lobe lesions remain a matter of speculation. The finding of a temporal gradient would support an interpretation based on progressive impairment of memory storage over a long period, whereas the finding that providing cues improves remote memory is compatible with a faulty retrieval hypothesis (Marslen-Wilson and Teuber, 1975).

Invoking a temporal gradient in retrograde amnesia assumes that the acquisition of information about the past events in question is temporally contiguous with their occurrence. However, the assumption is questionable (Squire and Slater, 1975). Conversely, recently acquired historical information may account for recall of past events. Variation in the level of item difficulty across time periods and cultural variation in following the news have also complicated attempts to use public events and photographs in evaluating remote memory. Squire and Slater (1975) employed a multiple choice questionnaire assessing recognition of the names of the television programs shown for a single season. They contended that incidental exposure to television shows was more common among Americans than exposure to newspapers and magazines. They also presented evidence to support the assumption that information tested on the television questionnaire is acquired close to the time when the show was broadcast.

Levin, Grossman, and Kelly (1977b) modified the television questionnaire of Squire and Slater for use with a young adult and teenage population by deleting the oldest programs. The protocol consisted of 32 questions that were equally divided among four time periods: 1966–1967, 1968–1969, 1970–1971, 1972–1973. A group of 28 adult patients with unequivocal evidence of brain damage (including 12 closed head injury patients and one patient with a left temporal gunshot wound) and a control group of medical patients without brain damage who were equivalent in age and education were compared. The pattern of results (Figure 4-2) showed marked impairment of retrograde memory in the brain-damaged group with no sparing of the most remote information. The data on the head-injured patients were analyzed separately to determine whether an acute onset of a brain lesion would produce a temporal gradient of retrograde amnesia not found in patients with insidious development of cerebral disease (e.g., neoplasm). Storage of information about television programs antedating the ictus in head-injured patients presumably should have been more resistant to retrograde amnesia. It was found that retention of the TV shows was comparable in the head-injured patients and in the cases with brain damage. The profiles of retrograde memory across time periods were also similar.

Recent studies by Squire and Slater (1978) suggest that a recall technique that probes for details of TV shows and public events is more likely to yield a temporal gradient than a multiple choice format. Consequently, it may be fruitful to apply the recall method to assessing retrograde amnesia in head-injured patients. The inclusion of very recent public events and TV program tests in the probe would permit evaluation of memory for information exposed to the patient shortly before injury. This technique is less useful with patients who rarely view TV and do not stay informed about news events.

Autobiographical memory

Cognitive psychologists have adopted a variant of Francis Galton's (1879) method of unconstrained search, which Galton had used to sample his own store of episodic memories to study recall of events in the life history. His method consisted of inspecting a word until an association was made to an event from his past followed by an attempt to date the memory. The results of subsequent

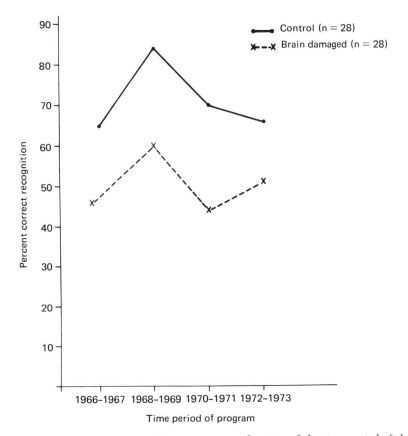

Fig. 4-2. Percent correct recognition memory as a function of the time period of the television program. [From Levin, H.S. et al. (1977). Assessment of long-term memory in brain-damaged patients. *J. Consult. Clin. Psychol. 45*:684–688. Reproduced with permission of the publisher.]

studies have consistently shown that the frequency of memories elicited decreases linearly as a function of their age (Crovitz and Quina-Holland, 1976; Franklin and Holding, 1977; Robinson, 1976). This pattern, which is opposite to that which would be predicted from Ribot's law, has been found in both young and elderly adults (Franklin and Holding, 1977). Serial administration of this procedure to closed head injury patients emerging from posttraumatic amnesia might elucidate their gradient of retrograde amnesia.

Duration of posttraumatic amnesia
in relation to quality of recovery

Russell (1932) assessed the outcome of closed head injury in 200 patients admitted to the Edinburgh Royal Infirmary by obtaining followup interviews at least
six months after injury. He classified the surviving patients into three groups
according to their posttraumatic amnesia duration (which he designated at that
time as "unconsciousness") as determined by retrospective questioning when
the patient's orientation had improved. He found that the likelihood of residual
memory disturbance (but not headaches or dizziness) was directly related to
posttraumatic amnesia duration. He also reported that age was related to it in
that memory deficit was more prominent across various levels of posttraumatic
amnesia duration in patients more than 40 years old. Subsequent studies of
closed head injury in British servicemen established that the duration of posttraumatic amnesia was directly related to residual neurologic deficits including
anosmia, aphasia, a residual retrograde amnesia greater than 30 minutes, memory impairment, calculation defects, and motor deficit (Russell and Smith,
1961). In contrast, "non-organic reactions" (e.g., anxiety, depression, dizziness
without vertigo, and headache) were not related to posttraumatic amnesia
duration. As compared to groups of closed head injury patients admitted to the
Oxford Military Hospital for Head Injuries within three weeks of injury, cases
transferred to Oxford after a longer interval because of difficulties in rehabilitation more frequently showed signs of the posttraumatic syndrome (see Chapter 9).

Russell also investigated posttraumatic amnesia duration in relation to outcome after an interval of at least two years after injury. Table 4-1 summarizes
the findings in 1,324 closed head injury patients. The findings in patients with
intracranial hematoma, depressed fracture, or focal signs were separately analyzed to ensure greater homogeneity with respect to type of injury. As the table
shows, discharge from the service on the grounds of disability was directly
related to duration of posttraumatic amnesia. This relationship was evident for
patients transferred to Oxford during the early stage of recovery (Groups A and
B), but was less clear in the "chronic" patients, who frequently evidenced emotional sequelae (Group C).

A correspondence between the duration of posttraumatic amnesia and outcome has been demonstrated in civilian closed head injury patients by Jennett
(1976b). As indicated in Table 4-3, the percentage of patients with moderate or
severe disability (Glasgow Outcome Scale) increases threefold or more when
posttraumatic amnesia exceeds seven days as estimated by retrospective inter-

Table 4-3. Relation between duration of posttraumatic amnesia (PTA) and rating of recovery according to the Glasgow Outcome Scale

PTA duration (days)	n	Severe disability (%)	Moderate disability (%)	Good recovery (%)
<7	11	—	9	91
7–14	27	—	26	74
15–28	38	2	45	53
>28	63	32	57	11

From Jennett, B. (1976) *Journal of Neurology, Neurosurgery, and Psychiatry* 39:647–655. Reproduced with permission of the publisher.

view data. As was pointed out by Russell (1935) and as is evident in Tables 4-1 and 4-3, posttraumatic amnesia has limitations as a prognostic criterion. Some patients with prolonged posttramatic amnesia achieve a good recovery and permanent disability is found in some patients with a relatively brief posttraumatic amnesia even when cases of focal injury are excluded. In view of the diverse determinants of global outcome, it is possible that specific neuropsychological measures may show a stronger relationship to the duration of posttraumatic amnesia than does the Glasgow Outcome Scale.

Posttraumatic amnesia as a predictor of cognitive recovery

Our review of the research concerned with cognitive recovery after closed head injury (Chapter 6) discloses discrepancies with respect to the predictive efficacy of posttraumatic amnesia duration. Serial intellectual assessment with the WAIS in the Glasgow studies has shown that the prognostic significance of this index of injury severity is time-limited (Mandleberg, 1976; Mandleberg and Brooks, 1975). Posttraumatic amnesia has been found to correlate with residual Verbal IQ up to three months after injury and with Performance IQ as long as six to nine months after injury. In these studies, the amnesia was measured directly by daily questioning and estimated retrospectively only in more severely injured cases who were amnesic at the time of discharge from the hospital. On the other hand, long- term (e.g., 30 months) Verbal and Performance IQs were unrelated to posttraumatic amnesia duration, although it should be noted that the IQ scores at this point in recovery were comparable to that of a control group.

More positive results have emerged from studies using retrospective measurement of posttraumatic amnesia and long-term followup. Von Wowern

(1966) reported that the percentage of patients with "moderate or severe dementia" two years after injury increased nearly twofold when posttraumatic amnesia was longer than seven days as compared to one to seven days. It is unclear how the presence of dementia was evaluated in this study. Further support for a relationship between posttraumatic amnesia duration and cognitive ability was provided by Norrman and Svahn (1961) who reported a significant correlation with Kohs Block Designs performance two years after injury. Roberts (1980) found that Raven's Progressive Matrices scores were lower in patients who had posttraumatic amnesia exceeding one week as compared to patients with briefer periods of amnesia when they were tested at least ten years after injury.

Greater agreement with respect to the predictive value of posttraumatic amnesia duration has been obtained in investigations of memory in the postamnesic period of recovery. However, these studies have not included serial testing as in the WAIS investigations at the University of Glasgow. Brooks (1975) found that scores on portions of the Wechsler Memory Scale were inversely related to the duration of posttraumatic amnesia (see Chapter 5). Visual memory deficit was also found by Brooks (1972) to be related to posttraumatic amnesia duration, which was estimated retrospectively. Accuracy in drawing a complex design from memory and continuous recognition memory for a series of recurring and nonrecurring line drawings were inversely related to the duration of the amnesia. The correlation between recognition memory performance and amnesia duration was more impressive for patients who were over 30 years old at the time of injury than for younger cases. Brooks et al. (1980) have reported that the retrospective estimate of posttraumatic amnesia duration is also related to verbal learning and retention and word fluency in closed head injury patients assessed within two years of injury.

Interpretation of the discrepancies in these studies is complicated by variation in the measurement of posttraumatic amnesia and the indices of cognitive function, as well as by such variables as the injury-test interval. It may be tentatively inferred from the Glasgow studies that the solution of novel visuospatial problems (e.g., Block Designs) and the capacity to learn and retain new information are more closely related to the duration of the amnesia than are abilities that more directly depend on previous education (e.g., Verbal IQ). In any case, the magnitude of the correlation between posttraumatic amnesia duration and residual cognitive ability has been rather modest and has rarely accounted for more than 25% of the variance in test scores. We are reminded of Russell's early findings showing that the type of injury (e.g., diffuse injury vs. mass lesion) affects the persistence of the amnesia. Future studies of the prognostic significance of posttraumatic amnesia should differentiate between diffuse closed head injury and injury with mass lesion. Direct quantitative assessment of the amnesia may provide a more useful index uncompromised by interobserver disagreement arising from nonstandardized procedure.

Memory function during posttraumatic amnesia

The question of whether patients have the capacity to store and retrieve information during posttraumatic amnesia has been raised by Schacter and Crovitz (1977). Although the learning and retention of information during such amnesia is, by definition, grossly impaired, there is ample evidence to suggest that residual memory function may be demonstrated by appropriate tests. This possibility is attested to by clinical reports of "islands of intact memory" during posttraumatic amnesia (Russell, 1932, 1935; Russell and Nathan, 1946). Apart from the theoretical import of determining the limits of information processing during the early phase of recovery, it is clinically significant with respect to the timing of physical therapy, speech therapy, and other rehabilitative procedures. As noted by Schacter and Crovitz, quantitative studies of cognitive function during the amnesic stage of recovery have failed to define posttraumatic amnesia according to an independent criterion (e.g., measures of orientation).

Schilder (1934) described the cognitive functioning of 35 closed head injury patients during the early stage of recovery and reported wide variation in memory test scores despite apparent posttraumatic amnesia in all cases. He found that recall of paragraphs read by the examiner and associative learning were markedly defective with relative sparing of "immediate memory" (digit span) and rote recall (e.g., counting). Ruesch and Moore (1943) found that serial subtraction was severely impaired in 120 closed head injury patients within the first 24 hours after injury. At the same time, they confirmed Schilder's finding of a relatively preserved digit span. As described in Chapter 6, studies in Glasgow have shown that closed head injury patients tested during posttraumatic amnesia obtain globally impaired scores on the WAIS, with a disproportionate deficit on the Performance Scale (Mandleberg, 1975).

More recently, Fodor (1972) investigated memory functions during posttraumatic amnesia in 47 closed head injury patients evaluated within 24 hours of injury. As in the earlier studies, no standard criterion for amnesia was employed. The sample was divided into "more or less severe injury" on the basis of whether IQ scores on a brief intelligence test were above or below 80. This procedure has been criticized on the grounds that it confounds premorbid intellectual ability with severity of injury (Schacter and Crovitz, 1977). Fodor found that immediate recall and recognition memory were preserved in the "less severe" group as was the delayed recall of unrelated test items. Recall of related items was, however, defective. In contrast, the "more severe" injury group exhibited a global memory deficit. Despite these methodologic deficiencies, Fodor's results suggest some capacity for learning and retention when patients are ostensibly amnesic following trauma.

Schacter and Crovitz (1977) have proposed some basic research questions for future studies of memory during posttraumatic amnesia. Drawing on data from studies of amnesic conditions other than head injury, they suggest that coding processes (e.g., auditory-verbal, visual) and cue utilization (e.g., semantic vs. phonemic) could be compared with the memory disorder in patients with Korsakoff's disease. Vulnerability to proactive interference, i.e., from material presented previously (Warrington and Weiskrantz, 1970), and the operation of storage and retrieval (Buschke and Fuld, 1974) could also be directly compared in closed head injury and Korsakoff patients. The relative preservation of motor skills despite anterograde amnesia in Korsakoff patients (Brooks and Baddeley, 1976) and after bimedial temporal lobectomy (Corkin, 1968) suggests that closed head injury patients might respond favorably to motor training even while they are amnesic. By extrapolation, it is conceivable that patients could transfer the gains made in physical therapy to the post-hospital environment even if they were amnesic for the total period of hospitalization.

Is learning during posttraumatic amnesia state dependent?

State dependent learning refers to the inability to retrieve information when testing is performed under a central state disparate from that which prevailed during learning. Weingartner (1978) postulated that incompatible strategies of encoding at the time of learning and later retrieval may underlie state dependent learning. Human state dependent learning has been primarily studied pharmacologically using a factorial design in which information is acquired during a drug (e.g., learning trials after alcohol ingestion) or non-drug state and later tested under a drug or non-drug state. Typically one-half of the subjects trained under a drug state are tested for retention under the same state and the other one-half are tested under a non-drug state. Subjects given initial training without drug administration are also divided into two states for testing retention, drug vs. non-drug. In general, performance (positive transfer) is superior in a congruent state (non-drug/non-drug; drug/drug) as compared with a non-congruent state (non-drug/drug; drug/non-drug). From his review of the literature, Weingartner concluded that the extent of state dependent learning depends upon the experimental task and the drug used. The strongest effects have been found in verbal learning and memory studies. Reversal of retrieval failure has been achieved by providing subjects with additional cues, suggesting that state dependent learning reflects inaccessibility to the contents of storage rather than erasure of information. Although most studies of dissociated human storage and retrieval states have used pharmacologically induced state dependent learning, transfer of training also has been investigated under altered mood states in patients with an affective disorder (Weingartner, Miller, and Murphy, 1977).

In view of the evidence for learning (however limited) during posttraumatic amnesia, a test of information transferred to the postamnesic period would determine whether state dependent learning is operating. If so, it may be possible to identify a physiologic discontinuity in brain state (e.g., changes in EEG, evoked potential, and cerebral blood flow) that differentiates the conditions of storage and retrieval.

Direct measurement of amnesia and disorientation

In the course of monitoring recovery of patients from closed head injury, clinicians regularly assess orientation in the post-comatose patient. Deterioration in cognitive level may be a sign of delayed hematoma or some other complication. This use of posttraumatic amnesia, which differs from Russell's emphasis on retrospective evaluation, provides information pertinent to treatment and planning for discharge. As noted by Russell and Nathan (1946), direct assessment of amnesia may be complicated by "islands of intact memory" during a period of confusion. Progressive shrinkage of retrograde amnesia is also likely to influence clinical judgment with respect to recovery. Clinical experience suggests that the conventional assessment of amnesia and disorientation can be appreciably affected by variation across examiners because there is no standardized procedure for measuring posttraumatic or retrograde amnesia.

Benton, Van Allen, and Fogel (1964) developed a brief quantitative test for temporal orientation, assessing the accuracy of a patient's knowledge of the day of the month, day of the week, month, year, and time. Points were deducted from a perfect score of 100 depending on the extent to which the patient's responses deviated from the correct answers on each question (see questions 6–10 in Figure 4-3). In a study of non-brain damaged patients (n 180) who were hospitalized on the neurologic, medical, and surgical services of University Hospitals, Iowa City, Levin and Benton (1975) found that nearly two-thirds of the patients had perfect test scores and only five patients (3%) had total scores less than 97 (four or more error points). In contrast, 13 (24%) of the 55 nonaphasic brain-damaged patients had scores below 97. As defined by this cutoff score, disorientation was associated with mental impairment and bilateral lesions, although it was not related to side of lesion when aphasics were excluded from the analysis. Although Benton, Van Allen, and Fogel (1964) found no relation between temporal orientation and educational level in neurologically normal patients, a recent study of normal adults residing in New Jersey (Natelson, Haupt, Fleischer, and Grey, 1979) indicated a small but statistically significant relationship between education and temporal orientation scores (above or below a criterion of 97). The major discontinuity was between subjects without a high school diploma and those who had completed high school. This study corroborated the findings of the Iowa studies showing that neurologists tend to overestimate the frequency of defects in temporal orientation in normal persons, i.e., are too liberal in estimating the lower limit of normal, particularly for individuals with at least a high school education. Extrapolation of these findings would suggest that clinicians are likely to underestimate the duration of posttraumatic amnesia, a trend previously noted by Russell (1935).

Levin, O'Donnell, and Grossman (1979) developed a brief schedule of questions to measure directly amnesia and disorientation after head injury. As shown in Figure 4-3, the temporal orientation questions used in the Iowa studies are included in the Galveston Orientation and Amnesia Test (GOAT). The GOAT asks the patient his name, address, and birthdate (Question 1) because patients recovering from severe closed head injury are often confused about basic biographic data and this information can usually be verified. Asking the patient to state the city or town he is in and to identify the building as a hospital (Question 2) probes for possible geographic disorientation and reduplication. Recall of the date of hospital admission (Question 3) was included because it was assumed that most patients are inclined to obtain this information, which is verifiable. Questions 4 and 5 probe events after and prior to the injury, respectively. Although the total GOAT score is interpreted as a global index of amnesia and disorientation, inclusion of these questions permits separate estimates of posttraumatic and retrograde amnesia as conventionally defined.

After entering the error points for each question, the sum is deducted from 100, yielding the total GOAT score (Figure 4-3). Instructions for scoring and a sample GOAT form are provided in Appendix B. It is advisable to administer the examination at least once a day. It can be administered when the vital signs are recorded. The graph of serial GOAT scores provides a clear record of recovery independently of such terms as "obtunded," "stuporous," or "disoriented," which may reflect interexaminer variation.

Name _____

Age _____ Sex M F

Date of Birth _____
mo day yr

Diagnosis _____

Date of Test |___|___|___|
mo day yr

Day of the week s m t w th f s

Time ___ AM PM

Date of injury |___|___|___|
mo day yr

GALVESTON ORIENTATION & AMNESIA TEST (GOAT)

Harvey S. Levin, Ph.D., Vincent M. O'Donnell, M.A., & Robert G. Grossman, M.D.

INSTRUCTIONS: Error points (shown in parentheses after each question) are scored for incorrect answers and are entered in the two columns on the extreme right side of the test form. Enter the total error points accrued for the 10 items in the lower right hand corner of the test form. The GOAT score equals 100 minus the total error points. Recovery of orientation is depicted by plotting serial GOAT scores on at least a daily basis.

Error Points

1. What is your name? (2) _____ When were you born? (4) _____

   Where do you live? (4) _____

2. Where are you now? (5) city _____ (5) hospital _____
   (unnecessary to state name of hospital)

3. On what date were you admitted to this hospital? (5) _____

   How did you get here? (5) _____

4. What is the first event you can remember after the injury? (5) _____

   Can you describe in detail (e.g., date, time, companions) the first event you can recall after injury? (5) _____

5. Can you describe the last event you recall before the accident? (5) _____

   Can you describe in detail (e.g., date, time, companions) _____

   the first event you can recall before the injury? (5) _____

6. What time is it now? _____ (1) for each ½ hour removed from correct time to maximum of 5)

7. What day of the week is it? _____ (1) for each day removed from correct one)

8. What day of the month is it? _____ (1) for each day removed from correct date to maximum of 5)

9. What is the month? _____ (5) for each month removed from correct one to maximum of 15)

10. What is the year? _____ (10) for each year removed from correct one to maximum of 30)

Total Error Points _____

Total GOAT Score (100-total error points) _____

Fig. 4-3. Questions comprising the Galveston Orientation and Amnesia Test (GOAT).

93

   The GOAT was standardized in a group of 50 predominantly young adults (median age 23) who had recovered from a mild closed head injury, i.e., momentary loss of consciousness or absence of coma, normal neurologic findings, and no obvious signs of confusion at the time of testing. This group was selected because it was demographically representative of the severe closed head injury population (at least in Houston and Galveston) and most of the patients could relate questions 3 through 5 to their personal experience of a head injury.

   The distribution of GOAT scores in Table 4-4 indicates that more than one-half the mild closed head injury group had scores over 95. The score below the entire mild group ($\leq$ 65) was thus considered to be defective, whereas the range from 66 to 75 was designated as borderline (exceeded by 92% of the group). Item analysis disclosed that no patient failed to correctly state basic biographic information (question 1) or the year (question 10); misidentification of the month (2% of the series), or of the present location (4%), was rare in this series of mild injuries. More commonly, the responses of these patients deviated from the correct day of the month (48%), time of day (30%), and date of admission (40%). Although the patients who recovered from mild closed head injury had no difficulty in describing the first event after injury or the last event prior to injury, elaboration of details (e.g., companions, time) was often vague and therefore the scores on questions 4 and 5 frequently reflected partial credit. Within the constraints of an age limit of 50 years and a median educational level of 11 years, there was no effect of either of these variables on the GOAT scores. Concurrent ratings by two examiners who alternated in interviewing the patients showed that there was a high level of interobserver agreement in scoring.

Table 4-4. Distribution of GOAT scores in patients who recovered from mild closed head injury

Score	Frequency	Percent of group
96–100	23	46
91–95	6	12
86–90	6	12
81–85	7	14
76–80	4	8
71–75	1	2
66–70	3	6

From Levin, H.S., O'Donnell, V.M., and Grossman, R.G. (1979). *Journal of Nervous and Mental Disease* 167:675–684. Reproduced with permission of the publisher.

Table 4-5. Eye opening rating on Glasgow Coma Scale in relation to performance on GOAT°

Eye opening on admission	Duration of PTA on GOAT						Total
	0–1 d	4–7 d	8–14 d	15 d–1 mo	1–2 mos	>2 mos	
None	—	—	—	3	5	7	15
To pain/speech	1	1	2	1	—	—	5
Spontaneous	11	4	8	1	1	—	25

From Levin, H.S., O'Donnell, V.M., and Grossman, R.G. (1979) *Journal of Nervous and Mental Disease* 167:675–684. Reproduced with permission of the publisher.
° PTA, posttraumatic amnesia; d, days; mos, months.

Table 4-6. Best motor response on Glasgow Coma Scale in relation to performance on GOAT°

Motor response on admission	Duration of PTA on GOAT						Total
	0–1 d	4–7 d	8–14 d	15 d–1 mo	1–2 mos	>2 mos	
None	—	—	—	—	—	—	—
Extension	—	—	—	1	2	1	4
Flexion	—	—	1	1	0	3	5
Localizes	—	2	1	4	3	3	13
Obeys commands	13	4	9	3	1	—	30

From Levin, H.S., O'Donnell, V.M., and Grossman, R.G. (1979). *Journal of Nervous and Mental Disease* 167:675–684. Reproduced with permission of the publisher.
° PTA, posttraumatic amnesia; d, days; mos, months; localizes, flexion, extension, and none refer to the patient's best response to painful stimulation.

Validity of serial GOAT scores was established in a series of 52 young adult closed head injury patients (median age 21) whose neurologic condition at the time of admission was rated by the Glasgow Coma Scale (Tables 4-5, 4-6, and 4-7). The test was initially given when the patient was able to cooperate and the test was repeated until the score improved to a level consistently above 75, a score clearly within the normal range of the standardization group. Duration of posttraumatic amnesia was defined as the period during which the GOAT score was 75 or less.

Analysis of serial GOAT scores showed a median posttraumatic amnesia interval of 14 days. This series was divided on the basis of posttraumatic amnesia duration and the Glasgow Coma Scale ratings of patients with long durations (above median) were compared to those of cases with durations below the median. Of the patients who had prolonged posttraumatic amnesia, a greater proportion exhibited impaired eye opening when admitted to the hospital (Table 4-5), were unable to follow commands (Table 4-6), and had incompre-

Table 4-7. Best verbal response on Glasgow Coma Scale in relation to performance on GOAT°

Verbal response on admission	Duration of PTA on GOAT						
	0–1 d	4–7 d	8–14 d	15 d–1 mo	1–2 mos	>2 mos	Total
None	—	2	—	5	4	6	17
Incomp	—	1	1	1	—	—	3
Inapp/conf	4	3	6	2	2	—	17
Oriented	9	1	3	—	—	—	13

From Levin, H.S., O'Donnell, V.M., and Grossman, R.G. (1979) *Journal of Nervous and Mental Disease* 167:675–684. Reproduced with permission of the publisher.
°PTA, posttraumatic amnesia; d, days; mos, months; Inapp/conf, inappropriate (e.g., explicatives) or confused (disoriented, but coherent); Incomp, incomprehensible (e.g., moaning).

hensible or no speech when admitted (Table 4-7) as compared to patients who had relatively brief periods of amnesia. The association between duration of posttraumatic amnesia as measured by the GOAT and acute neurologic impairment was highly significant ($p < 0.0001$) for the eye, motor, and verbal components of the Glasgow Coma Scale. Levin, O'Donnell, and Grossman (1979) concluded that serial GOAT scores were strongly related to the severity of acute cerebral disturbance after closed head injury. In the same series, posttraumatic amnesia that persisted beyond two weeks was associated with CT findings indicative of diffuse closed head injury or bilateral lesions, whereas GOAT scores usually improved more rapidly in patients with focal mass lesions.

Long-term assessment of outcome at least six months after injury was completed in 32 of the patients. Overall social and vocational recovery was rated according to the Glasgow Outcome Scale (Jennett and Bond, 1975), which is described in Chapter 3. Table 4-8 shows that most patients with posttraumatic amnesia periods less than 2 weeks achieved a good recovery; longer intervals of

Table 4-8. Duration of posttraumatic amnesia on GOAT as a predictor of long-term outcome°

Long-term outcome	Duration of PTA on GOAT						
	0–1 d	4–7 d	8–14 d	15 d–1 mo	1–2 mos	>2 mos	Total
Good recovery	3	4	7	2	0	0	16
Mod/severe disability	—	—	1	5	5	5	16

From Levin, H.S., O'Donnell, V.M., and Grossman, R.G. (1979) *Journal of Nervous and Mental Disease* 167:675–684. Reproduced with permission of the publisher.
°PTA, posttraumatic amnesia; d, days; mos, months.

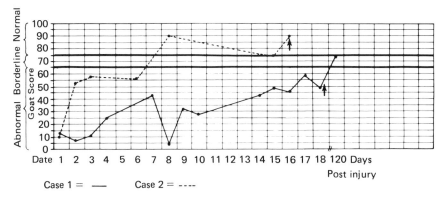

Fig. 4-4. Recovery curves of two patients on the Galveston Orientation and Amnesia Test (GOAT) during the initial hospitalization after severe closed head injury (Case 1) and mild injury (Case 2). The first date (*x* axis) begins on the day of admission (Case 2) and after four days of coma (Case 1).

amnesia were frequently followed by prolonged disability. From these findings we concluded that the GOAT is useful in characterizing the early phase of recovery in the noncomatose patient. This has proven to be particularly evident in patients who proceed from very brief periods of coma (i.e., one or two hours) to prolonged confusional states that fluctuate in the degree of disorientation, amnesia, and behavioral disturbance.

Figure 4-4 depicts GOAT recovery curves during the initial hospitalization for two cases of closed head injury. Successive dates (plotted on the *x* axis) begin with the first day that the patient was able to respond to commands and cooperate for Case 1. The graph begins on the day of admission for Case 2 because this was a patient with a mild injury who was never comatose. Both patients exhibited marked behavioral disturbance during the period in which the GOAT scores reflected severe disorientation and amnesia.

Case 1. A 24-year-old woman sustained a closed head injury in an automobile accident; upon arrival at the emergency room, her Glasgow Coma Scale score was 8, as she opened her eyes only to pain, localized to pain, and had no speech. Neurologic findings included a third nerve palsy and a sixth nerve underaction; her left pupil was nonreactive. A CT scan on the day of admission showed slit-like ventricles consistent with diffuse cerebral swelling. She responded to simple commands four days after the injury, but was markedly confused and agitated as evidenced by arm thrashing and by kicking. As the patient began to verbalize, she exhibited a florid psychosis marked by visual hallucinations and unsystematized delusions (e.g., she was hospitalized "to have a baby"). The patient's psychotic symptoms gradually resolved after two weeks; her GOAT recovery curve (Figure 4-4) indicates persistence of disorientation and amnesia throughout the period of hospitalization. Follow-up assessment four months after injury disclosed low normal orientation (Figure 4-4), although detailed neuropsychological studies revealed slowed reaction time and memory deficit. Eventually she achieved a good recovery after a year of moderate disability.

Case 2. This 21-year-old student sustained a closed head injury in an automobile accident and was initially evaluated at a local hospital where he was described as "comatose." Upon arrival at The University of Texas Medical Branch three hours after injury, the patient's eyes opened spontaneously, he responded to commands, but his verbalizations were inappropriate (Glasgow Scale score 13). Despite the apparently mild severity of the initial injury, he developed a posttraumatic psychosis that persisted for 10 days. Manifestations of the psychosis included visual and tactile hallucinations and fragmentary delusions. Autonomic activation was reflected by intermittent agitation and profuse sweating. Neurologic examination showed motor rigidity in all extremities, but was otherwise normal. A CT scan on the day of admission was normal. By comparison with Case 1, it can be seen (Figure 4-4) that his recovery curve rises more steeply to within the normal range prior to the time of discharge. As anticipated from the study of outcome, he was better prepared to resume activities of daily living during the immediate post-hospitalization period than was Case 1.

The findings reaffirmed the potential clinical significance of posttraumatic amnesia while supporting its direct measurement by a standardized method. Serial scores yielding a recovery curve have been shown to provide clinically useful, unambiguous information. Future studies might compare the results of posttraumatic amnesia estimated from retrospective data to that of serial GOAT scores. The correlation between coma duration (as indicated by the Glasgow Scale) and persistence of amnesia/confusion on the GOAT could also be studied to ascertain the possibility of a linear relationship.

Summary

Posttraumatic amnesia is a prominent feature of closed head injury. Its persistence varies with the type and severity of initial neurologic injury. Its direct serial measurement by standardized procedures can yield reliable information of prognostic significance for long- term recovery. The limits of learning and memory during posttraumatic amnesia remain unexplored as does the possibility of transfer of information to the post-amnesic state.

5. Memory function

Amnesia, whether anterograde or retrograde, has an acute onset and resolves at a varying rate. A residual memory deficit may persist after the amnesia clears, as shown in Figure 5-1, which depicts the various types of mnemonic disorder after head injury. In view of the pathophysiologic mechanisms of head injury discussed in Chapter 1 and the importance of the temporal lobes for mnemonic function, memory disorder is likely to be a prominent sequel of closed head injury. As has been noted, the temporal lobes are predisposed to focal contusion and hematoma by their structural irregularity and the bony protusion of the sphenoid wing (Gurdjian and Gurdjian, 1976). Moreover, bilateral shearing and tearing of fiber tracts within the temporal stem may disrupt afferent and efferent connections of the temporal cortex and the amygdala.

Following Schacter and Crovitz (1977), our discussion is divided into sections according to the stage of recovery, i.e., memory function during and immediately after posttraumatic amnesia and long-term recovery. As will be seen, investigators have not consistently reported the level of orientation at the time of memory testing; consequently, the differentiation of the posttraumatic amnesia stage and subsequent stages is not clear in some studies. However, the scope of our review has been broadened to include neurologic mechanisms in memory deficit, more recently published studies, and a description of newer methods and findings. Studies reporting only the frequency of complaints of memory deficit without the results of quantitative assessment or at least of a clinical mental status examination are not considered. Memory during posttraumatic amnesia is discussed in Chapter 4.

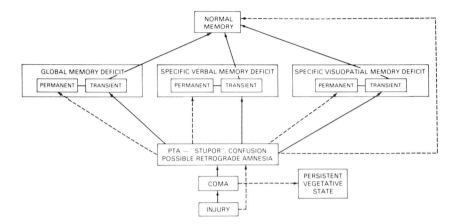

Fig. 5-1. Residual memory functioning after the subacute stage of recovery from closed head injury. Note that a material-specific or global memory deficit frequently persists for varying durations after resolution of posttraumatic amnesia (PTA), although no memory disturbance may be present following the brief period of PTA associated with minor head trauma.

Methodologic flaws in published studies of memory after closed head injury are similar to those discussed in the section on intellectual recovery. These include failure to screen for preexisting conditions (e.g., alcoholism) that potentially compromise memory, inadequate documentation of the severity of head injury and of the presence of mass lesions, and the use of nonuniform intervals between injury and assessment. A further complication in integrating these studies is the use of disparate measures of mnemonic function, which in part reflect continued debate among researchers concerning the basic processes of normal memory. Few memory tests now employed in clinical practice reflect recent advances in cognitive psychology and no memory test has achieved wide acceptance as a standard of measurement similar to the status of the WAIS in the assessment of adult intelligence.

In contrast to studies of intellectual recovery, there are no available means of obtaining preinjury baseline levels of specific memory abilities. Memory tests, unlike intellectual and academic achievement tests, are not used on a wide scale for screening purposes. To clarify the interpretation of memory findings vis-à-vis head injury severity, it is useful to exclude from the study patients with known preinjury cognitive defects and to differentiate between subgroups of closed head injury patients according to indices of severity. Testing uninjured normal subjects of similar age and assessing the memory of oriented closed head

injury patients who have recovered from mild head injury (i.e., with no neurologic deficit or loss of consciousness persisting beyond a few minutes) also
increases our confidence in identifying unequivocal memory impairment. The
mild closed head injury comparison group should be comprised of individuals
with a demographic background similar to that of the more severe injuries; for-
tuitous circumstances (e.g., seating position) often determine which occupants
of a vehicle suffer the least severe injuries. As will be seen, mild head injury
may produce a transient memory deficit that resolves by the time of followup.

Memory function after recovery of orientation

In contrast to the boundary between posttraumatic amnesia and normal orientation suggested by the stages of memory recovery depicted in Figure 4-1 and
implicit in earlier studies, most investigators have failed to clearly define the
criteria for inferring termination of posttraumatic amnesia. Where no opera-
tional definition has been applied, it is advisable to view critically distinctions
that are made between resolving memory deficit during and soon after posttraumatic amnesia. Schacter and Crovitz (1977) have commented on the lack
of physiologic or biochemical studies pertinent to the issue of whether termination of posttraumatic amnesia marks a biologic threshold in the recovery process. Notwithstanding the foregoing reservations, it may be noted that there is
general agreement in the literature that a residual memory deficit of varying
duration is common after posttraumatic amnesia however it is defined.

Frequency of memory deficit
after posttraumatic amnesia termination

Reports of memory deficit based on large series of patients suggest that it is a
very frequent sequel of closed head injury. In several articles and monographs,
Russell and coworkers (Russell, 1932, 1971; Russell and Smith, 1961) depicted
the frequency of "memory and/or calculation defect" in British soldiers who
sustained nonpenetrating head injury during World War II and were transferred to the Oxford Military Hospital for Head Injuries. The data were derived
from the results of examinations by a staff that included neurologists, neurosurgeons, and psychologists, but the procedures utilized for the assessment of memory are not specified in the published papers. Of 1,324 closed head injury
patients (432 cases with depressed skull fracture, intracranial complication, or
severe extracranial injury were analyzed separately), Russell (1971) reported
some degree of memory deficit in 310 (23%) of the sample. The proportion of

patients who evidenced residual memory deficit was closely related to the duration of posttraumatic amnesia, with more than one-half of the patients with posttraumatic amnesia exceeding seven days being affected.

Immediate (short-term) memory after posttraumatic amnesia termination

Research findings on cognitive processes in normal subjects and findings from clinical studies of memory disturbances have converged to differentiate two memory systems. Immediate or short-term memory, frequently referred to as "primary" or "working memory" (Watkins, 1974; Wickelgreen, 1975), is a limited capacity system that holds approximately seven chunks of information over periods of less than a minute. Information in short-term memory is highly vulnerable to displacement by subsequently presented stimuli and distraction. Whereas various experimental paradigms, such as the Brown-Peterson technique (Peterson and Peterson, 1959), have gained wide acceptance as measures of short-term memory, classification of the digit span test continues to be disputed among memory theorists. In the literature of clinical neuropsychology and neurology, digit span is generally regarded as a measure of short-term memory. Persuasive neurologic evidence supporting the operation of two distinct memory systems has come from studies of patients with generalized amnesic disorder secondary to Wernicke-Korsakoff disease, herpes simplex encephalitis, and bilateral temporal lobe surgical resection. In contrast to marked impairment in learning and retention of new information that exceeds the capacity of memory span, patients with generalized memory disorder frequently exhibit a normal or near normal digit span. In a young woman with a residual amnesic disorder following herpes simplex encephalitis, Peters and Levin (1977) found remarkable preservation of auditory digit span (8 digits forward, 7 digits backward), despite a Wechsler Memory Quotient of 73. Accordingly, relative preservation of digit span might be anticipated after closed head injury. Greater sparing of forward span would be expected insofar as reversing digits demands a strategy of auditory or visual rehearsal and more persistent retention that presumably activate long-term memory processes.

Ruesch (1944b) serially tested digit span in 53 closed head injury admissions to the Boston City Hospital. Within 24 hours of admission, the mean forward and backward spans were 5.8 and 3.6, respectively, in this series of cases that were heterogeneous in severity. Reexamination four to 12 weeks after injury disclosed only minor improvement with a mean forward span of 6.2 and a mean backward span of 4.0. Differentiation of the patients according to whether their performance improved (n 25) or remained stationary (n 28) disclosed that impaired digit span was relatively infrequent on the initial examination, even in the "stationary" group and was nonexistent by the time of the final test in patients who generally improved. Relatively unimpaired and stable immediate recall on digit span was confirmed by Fodor (1972), who also tested patients within 24 hours of injury and studied them serially for several days. Consistent with the possibility of the relative preservation of immediate memory, Cronholm and Jonsson (1957) found no significant difference in digit span between 20 closed head injury patients who were unconscious for no more than a few minutes and a control group, when the head-injured patients were tested about one week after injury. By comparison, administration of the WAIS to relatively mild closed head injury patients shortly after admission and again ten weeks later was found by Becker (1975) to produce a significant improvement in digit span that was not found in control subjects tested repeatedly. In agreement with Becker's findings, the Glasgow studies have shown impairment of digit span during posttraumatic amnesia with significant improvement when the initial level was compared to scores up to three years after injury (Mandleberg, 1975, 1976; Mandleberg and Brooks, 1975). Of the verbal subtests of the WAIS, only the digit span scores of closed head injury patients differed from those of a control group when the former were evaluated three years postinjury.

Assessment of digit span in normally oriented closed head injury patients was investigated by Brooks (1972) in a wider study of the Wechsler Memory Scale in which patients with closed head injury of varying severity were tested at different intervals after injury. The author reported that the forward span of closed head injury patients was comparable to that of control subjects, whereas the backward span was significantly impaired. A dissociation of forward–backward span was also shown in an analysis of posttraumatic amnesia duration, since this variable was related only to subsequent backward span. Thomsen (1977) found that auditory digit span was still reduced more than two years after severe head injury in patients with residual aphasia, but it had recovered to a normal level in nonaphasic closed head injury cases.

Short-term visual memory after closed head injury was investigated by Levin, Grossman, and Kelly (1976), who tested recognition of irregularly shaped designs immediately after a 10-sec presentation. Despite pretest screening to ensure normal or greatly improved orientation, the patients with closed head injury complicated by protracted coma or oculovestibular deficit evidenced impaired short-term visual memory when tested at long intervals after injury.

Interpretation of these disparate reports would suggest that immediate memory, as reflected by forward digit span, is comparatively resistant to the effects of closed head injury. Mildly injured patients may display no evidence of reduced forward span even when tested early after admission. Although digit span is disturbed in the early stages of recovery from more severe injury, persistent deficit is primarily confined to backward span and short-term visual memory. The degree to which immediate memory is compromised by closed head injury may depend on the format of information such that immediate recall for numbers is less impaired than is short-term recognition memory for complex designs.

Wechsler Memory Scale

Clinical psychologists frequently administer the Wechsler Memory Scale (Wechsler and Stone, 1945) to assess memory deficit in patients with known or suspected brain damage. Although the test has been criticized on methodologic grounds and is obsolete in view of the experimental procedures developed by cognitive psychologists (Erickson and Scott, 1977), Brooks (1975) found that subtests of the Wechsler Memory Scale were indeed sensitive to the effects of closed head injury when patients were tested after unequivocal resolution of posttraumatic amnesia. Justifiably objecting to Wechsler's convention of summing the raw scores of subtests that measure different processes to obtain a composite score, Brooks discarded the memory quotient in his study of 82 closed head injury patients who were heterogeneous in injury severity, age (16 to 60), and the injury-test interval (same day as injury to 24 months after injury). In comparison with a control group of 34 orthopedic patients, the closed head injury group was more impaired on general information (e.g., name of President), orientation, recall of brief stories presented orally, verbal paired associates, reversal of digits, and reproduction of visual designs after a 10-sec presentation. Posttraumatic amnesia duration was also inversely related to performance on these tests. In contrast, rote recall of overlearned sequences (e.g., alphabet) and digits forward did not differentiate the groups nor was duration of amnesia strongly related to these variables. A similar pattern emerged when the closed head injury patients were grouped according to grades of severity based on neurologic findings and overall outcome. Brooks supplemented the standard procedure by testing delayed recall of the stories one hour later. Unexpectedly, the decrement in delayed vs. immediate recall was not disproportionately greater in the closed head injury patients, although the level of initial performance was not matched for the two groups.

From these findings, it may be inferred that the Wechsler Memory Scale is useful for clinical evaluation of closed head injury, although it is clearly advisable for clinicians to obtain normative data for non-head–injured patients of similar demographic background if an analysis of subtest scores is contemplated. The pattern of findings is compatible with increased vulnerability of intermediate memory after closed head injury with relative sparing of short-term (immediate) memory and the recall of sequences overlearned prior to injury.

Long-term memory after posttraumatic amnesia termination

The extensive literature on the memory disorders associated with Korsakoff's syndrome in alcoholics (Butters and Cermak, 1980), surgical lesions of the medial temporal lobes (Scoville and Milner, 1957), and herpes simplex encephalitis (Drachman and Arbit, 1966) indicates that learning and retention of new information are impaired, whereas immediate memory may be relatively preserved. Depending on the paradigms used by various investigators, the observed long-term memory deficit in amnesic patients has been attributed to deficient retrieval from long-term storage (Warrington and Weiskrantz, 1968), defective encoding that results in inadequate self-cuing (Cermak and Butters, 1972), and reduced capacity for long-term storage. In contrast to numerous studies of Korsakoff's snydrome, relatively few quantitative investigations have explored the processes most affected in closed head injury patients with deranged memory.

The distinction between short- and long-term memory was investigated by Brooks (1975) in a study in which patients were asked to recall a list of words in any order ("free recall") immediately after presentation in a fixed order on repeated trials. Findings on this task in normal subjects characteristically show a "recency effect" in which the probability of recall is highest for the terminal items and decreases rapidly the further an item is from the end of the list, although retention of words from the initial portion of the list is usually somewhat better than the middle portion. Recall from the latter portion of the word list is presumed to reflect short-term memory, whereas it is supposed that long-term memory mediates recall from the initial portion of the list because of the longer retention interval and the necessity for a more permanent form of storage (cf. Baddeley, 1976). The relatively low probability of recall of words from the middle portion of the list is attributed to less efficient long-term storage and interference from both earlier and later words. Although the necessity for invoking the operation of two memory systems to explain the recency effect in free recall has drawn criticism (Wickelgreen, 1975), evidence for a dissociation comes from a study of Korsakoff patients by Baddeley and Warrington (1970) in which the magnitude of memory deficit was greatest for words at the beginning of the list (long-term memory component) and retention was relatively unimpaired for words in the latter portion of the list (short-term memory component).

Brooks (1975) tested free recall for word lists in 30 patients with closed head injury of varying severity (posttraumatic amnesia < 24 hours to > 40 days) who ranged in age from 15 to 60 years. As shown in Figure 5-2, the portion of the performance curve corresponding to words at the beginning of the list (long-term memory) shows a greater disparity between the closed head injury patients and control group as compared to the later section of the curve that represents recall of words toward the end of the list (short-term memory). Despite the trend evident in Figure 5-2, group differences were not confirmed for either portion of the curve.

More impressive results were found when Brooks assessed long-term memory in both groups by imposing a 20-sec delay between presentation of the word list

Fig. 5-2. Mean percentage of correct recall as a function of word position for closed head-injured and control patients with recall tested immediately after presentation of the words. [From Brooks, D.N. (1975). Long- and short-term memory in head-injured patients. *Cortex, 11*:329–340.]

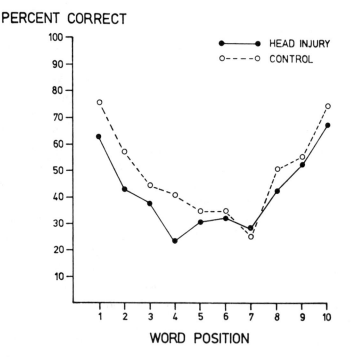

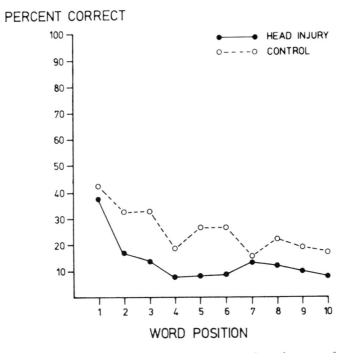

Fig. 5-3. Mean percentage of correct recall as a function of word position for head-injured and control patients, delayed recall. [From Brooks, D.N. (1975). Long- and short-term memory in head-injured patients. *Cortex, 11*:329–340.]

and recall; the patient was asked to count backwards during the interpolated interval to prevent rehearsal of the words. Delayed recall with distraction by a subsidiary activity had been shown previously to abolish the recency effect on this task in normal subjects (Glanzer and Cunitz, 1966), presumably by disrupting the transfer of information from short-term memory to more permanent storage and displacing items from short-term memory because of demands imposed by counting backwards. Under the delay condition (Fig. 5-3), recall by closed head injury patients was significantly below that of the control group.

Brooks further analyzed short- and long-term memory components in free recall, using the Tulving and Colotla (1970) classification of each word on a basis of the number of intervening presentations and recalls of other words (retention interval) on a trial. A retention value of 7 or less was defined as short-term memory, and an interval of 8 or more was defined as long-term memory. Applying these definitions, Brooks found no difference between closed head injury patients and the control group on the number of items in short-term memory, whereas a comparison of items in the long-term memory barely reached significance. The author buttressed his interpretation of these findings by showing that the two groups did not differ in digit span, a putative measure of short-term memory. He inferred that impaired storage was the basis for defective long-term memory in the head-injured patients because they had fewer errors of intrusion from previous word lists (which would suggest disturbed retrieval) than control subjects. However, in their review, Schacter and Crovitz contend that the absence of intrusions from other lists is not convincing evidence for implicating a storage deficit.

Clinical observation indicates that closed head injury patients with severe memory deficit sometimes intrude items in a broader sense, e.g., the names of objects in the examining room and aspects of the hospital environment may find their way into the patient's recall (Weinstein and Kahn, 1955). Consistent with these observations, Brooks found that extralist errors occurred more frequently in the protocols of closed head injury patients than in the control group and that semantic confusion between the test word and intrusion predominated over acoustic errors. He cited previous studies of normal memory, suggesting that semantic coding predominates in transferring information into permanent storage to support his view that long-term memory was primarily impaired in closed head injury patients. More recent studies, however, have shown that various codes are available to short- and long-term stages of memory and that the acoustic–semantic dichotomy may be an artifact of specific test procedures (Watkins, 1974). Of the findings obtained by Brooks, the potentiation of group differences by delaying recall with a distractor task probably constitutes the most persuasive evidence for the short-term–long-term memory dissociation. It is conceivable that the selection of a group of closed head injury cases more homogeneous in respect to severity of injury would result in a sharper contrast between short- and long-term memory.

Buschke and Fuld (1974) developed a selective reminding procedure that is adjustive and thus efficient for use with brain-damaged patients. In contrast to conventional verbal memory tests, the examiner presents on each successive trial only those items the patient missed on the preceding trial. The selective reminding procedure is similar to the adjustive version of the Supraspan Test (Drachman and Arbit, 1966) in which the patient's capacity to add to his forward span (the longest series of digits prior to two consecutive failures) is tested over repeated trials. Recall of an item in the absence of its presentation is interpreted by Buschke as evidence for encoding into long-term storage. After entering long-term storage, information about an item may be retrieved consistently without the necessity for additional reminders, or retrieval failure might occur with a varying probability.

Figure 5-4A (cf. 5-4B) depicts the selective reminding results of a normal high school student who was given a slightly modified version of the test used by Buschke. The items are words that occur frequently in English usage, as inferred from the American Heritage Word Frequency Book (Carroll, Davies, and Richman, 1971). Long-term storage, i.e., recall of a word on at least one trial without it being presented, is denoted by the thick underline. Consistent retrieval of the item, i.e., recall with no additional reminding, is designated by the arrow on the first trial of an uninterrupted recall series. The scoring section on the lower portion of the figure includes several other variables. Short-term recall refers to recall dependent on presentation of the item, i.e., without evidence of storage. Long-term retrieval includes both consistent and random retrieval (variable retrieval of word across trials after it has entered storage). Total recall on a trial is the sum of words recalled from short- and long-term retrieval.

Administration of the selective reminding test to a group of 50 high school students in Galveston disclosed an impressive rate of acquisition as reflected by consistent retrieval of most words midway through the procedure. Reminding was rarely needed after a few trials. In accord with developmental studies of memory (Maccoby and Jacklin, 1974) that suggest that girls are more proficient in verbal memory than boys, long-term retrieval in female students surpassed that in males. The finding of female superiority on the selective reminding task has since been corroborated in college students by Hannay (personal communication). Consequently, it was necessary to establish the cutoff for the lower limit of the normal range separately for each sex.

In a recent application of Buschke's selective reminding procedure to assess long-term memory, Levin and Eisenberg (1979c) classified 96 young adult and adolescent closed head injury patients (median age 20 years) into groups according to whether their injury was mild, diffuse, complicated by a lateralized mass effect, or associated with a bilateral mass lesion. Participation in this study was confined to patients with no evidence of an antecedent condition that would place them at risk for memory deficit. To determine the maximum frequency of memory deficit after resolution of posttraumatic amnesia, the analysis was based on the initial assessment (within six months of injury) after the patient's orientation had improved to within normal limits on the GOAT or at least had reached a stable plateau of recovery (median 23 days). Accordingly, mildly injured patients were tested after a relatively brief interval (median 16 days), whereas assessment of patients with diffuse (median 42 days) or bilateral mass

NAME: CONTROL ♂   DATE: 3-76

AGE: 17   EDUC.: 11

SELECTIVE REMINDING

	1	2	3	4	5	6	7	8	9	10	11	12
Bowl	1		2▷	1	5	3	11	3	10	3	12	1
Passion	2▷	5	6	6	8	2	2	8	6	9	7	6
Dawn		4▷	9	7	9	9	3	7	7	6	8	5
Judgement	5▷	2	5	8	7	7	4	6	5	11	6	7
Grant			1▷	3	4	5	7	5	3	5	11	2
Bee		6▷	7	10	10	10	6	12	1	2	10	10
Plane	6▷	1	8	9	11	8	10	10	8	10	9	9
County	4	8	11	11	2	11		1▷	9	7	3	11
Choice			3		1▷	6	8	2	2	8	4	12
Seed	3▷	7	10	4	12	1	5	9	12	1	2	8
Wool		3	12	5	6		1▷	11	11	12	1	4
Meal			4▷	2	3	4	9	4	4	4	5	3
Total Recall	6	8	12	11	12	11	11	12	12	12	12	12
LTR	5	8	11	11	12	11	11	12	12	12	12	12
STR	1	0	1	0	0	0	0	0	0	0	0	0
LTS	5	8	11	11	12	12	12	12	12	12	12	12
CLTR	4	6	9	9	10	10	11	12	12	12	12	12
Random LTR	1	2	2	2	2	1	0	0	0	0	0	0
Presentations	12	6	4	0	1	0	1	1	0	0	0	0

LTR = LONG TERM RETRIEVAL
STR = SHORT TERM RECALL
LTS = LONG TERM STORAGE
CLTR = CONSISTENT LONG TERM RETRIEVAL
RANDOM LTR = RANDOM LONG TERM RETRIEVAL

Fig. 5-4A. Selective reminding test protocol of a normal high school student. Long-term storage of words is denoted by underline; arrows indicate the beginning of consistent retrieval from long-term storage, i.e., retrieval without the necessity of further reminding. The numbers indicate the order in which the words were recalled on each trial. Absence of underline indicates that recall of a word was dependent on its presentation.

injury (median 31 days) was frequently delayed by protracted coma or confusion.

Mild closed head injury (n 46) was defined as an injury that produced either no loss of consciousness or a coma persisting no longer than a few minutes at the time of impact, normal neurologic findings, and normal CT images when this radiologic study was performed. Lateralized mass effect was defined by the presence of a unilateral intracranial hematoma, contusion, or focal edema as demonstrated by CT (although in several patients injured prior to 1975, the results of angiography were used). On this basis, 11 patients with left hemisphere mass lesion and ten right hemisphere cases were identified, although this designation in no way precluded concomitant diffuse effects. There were five cases with bilateral mass lesions. Diffuse closed head injury (n 24) was inferred when coma persisted beyond a few minutes in a patient with no evidence of mass effect. In agreement with previous analyses of CT in diffuse injury (Zimmerman and Bilaniuk, 1979), the authors distinguished between diffuse injury

Fig. 5-4B. Initial selective reminding protocol (9 days after injury) after surgical removal of a left temporal epidural hematoma. The patient was oriented and nonaphasic at the time of testing. Note the marked impairment of consistent retrieval. Retesting 11 months later showed marked improvement well within the normal range of high school students.

SELECTIVE REMINDING TEST

NAME: ♂ CHI   DATE: 8-1-78

AGE: 14   EDUCATION: 8

DIAGNOSIS: LEFT TEMPORAL HEMATOMA

MULT CH

	1	2	3	4	5	6	7	8	9	10	11	12		CR	L	R
BOWL				9		1	8					1	BOWL	*	Ac	bd
PASSION	1		6	4		3	5	5		7◄	3	5	PASSION		ac	bD
DAWN				2			1				1		DAWN		Ac	bd
JUDGEMENT			3	4		3	4		2◄	4	6		JUDGE-MENT	*	aC	bd
GRANT				7	6	9	8	7	8			2	GRANT	*	ac	Bd
BEE	3	3	5	5	6	5		2◄	5	6	6	9	BEE	■	ac	bD
PLANE			2	7			2		1◄	4	8	8	PLANE	*	ac	Bd
COUNTY			1	4	8	5	8		3		1	7	COUNTY	*	Ac	bd
CHOICE			3		3		4		2◄	3	5	7	CHOICE	*	aC	bd
SEED	2	2		2	1	4	7	6	4	5		3	SEED	*	ac	Bd
WOOL				1		2	1		3			4	WOOL	*	aC	bd
MEAL			1	6		7	6	7	6		2		MEAL	*	ac	bD
													TOTALS	9	12	

INTRUSIONS

TOTAL INTRU-SIONS 2	BULL	BULL										

	1	2	3	4	5	6	7	8	9	10	11	12
Σ RECALL	3	3	6	9	7	8	9	8	7	8	8	9
LTR	2	3	5	7	5	8	8	7	7	8	7	9
STR	1	0	1	2	2	0	1	1	0	0	1	0
LTS	2	3	6	7	8	10	10	10	11	11	11	11
CLTR	0	0	0	0	0	0	0	1	3	5	5	5
RLTR	2	3	5	7	5	8	8	6	4	3	2	4
REMINDERS	12	9	9	6	3	5	4	3	4	5	4	4

COMMENTS

30' RECALL

PLANE
MEAL
SEED
BEE
COUNTY
CHOICE
PASSION

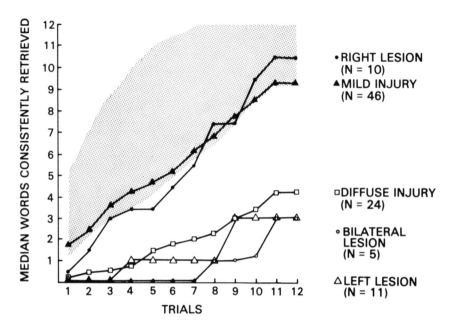

Fig. 5-5. Consistent retrieval from long-term storage plotted across trials for initial test-ing (mean injury-test interval, 40 days) after recovery of orientation. The subgroups of closed head injury designated left, right, and bilateral refer to the lateralization of mass lesion by CT, whereas diffuse injury implies the absence of hematoma, contusion, or focal edema. Mild injury implies momentary or no loss of consciousness and normal neurologic findings. Shaded area depicts retrieval by normal adolescents (± 1 S.D.).

associated with normal images (n 4) and a subgroup in which the lateral ven-tricles were obscured or "slit-like," suggesting compression by cerebral swelling (n 11). In this series CT was not performed in nine diffuse closed head injury patients.

Consistent retrieval of words across trials is depicted for each closed head injury group in Figure 5-5; there is a trend for relatively preserved verbal learn-ing and memory in patients with mild closed head injury and patients with right hemisphere mass lesions. Summing the number of words consistently retrieved on each trial yielded total retrieval scores that were used to compare the groups. Application of the Mann–Whitney Test disclosed that consistent retrieval by patients with mild closed head injury surpassed that of the left mass lesion group ($p < 0.01$), the diffuse closed head injury patients ($p < 0.0001$), and the bilateral group ($p < 0.05$). Apart from the contrasts involving the mild head-injured group, the difference in retrieval between the right hemisphere group and the diffuse injury patients only approached significance ($p < 0.06$). Not shown here are the findings for long-term storage, which corresponded closely to those of retrieval.

Analysis of focal CT findings showed that a circumscribed mass lesion was situated in the left temporal lobe in five cases; the remaining five left hemisphere patients had mass lesions primarily in the frontal and parietal lobes, although in three of these patients, there was extension into the temporal lobe. Further analysis suggested that left temporal injury was the primary contributing factor to the overall deficit in the left hemisphere group. Patients with a left hemisphere mass lesion that did not primarily infiltrate the temporal lobe evidenced storage and retrieval comparable to that of the right hemisphere cases. In support of these trends, total consistent retrieval in the left temporal lesion patients was significantly below that of the left nontemporal patients ($p < 0.004$) and the right hemisphere patients ($p < 0.05$). Findings on storage also implicated the grave consequences of left temporal mass lesion for memory. Figure 5-4B depicts the initial selective reminding protocol of a patient who had a left temporal epidural hematoma surgically removed before base-line testing. Impaired retrieval of information in storage was evident, whereas multiple choice recognition was errorless. An unannounced recall trial 30 minutes after the test disclosed retention of seven words as compared to recall of at least ten words in normal adolescents.

The frequency of unequivocal storage and retrieval deficit is shown for each closed head injury group in Table 5-1. Fisher's exact method disclosed that the relative frequency of storage and/or retrieval deficit was greater in patients

Table 5-1. Defective storage and retrieval in relation to severity and type of closed head injury°

| Memory deficit | Mild (n 46) | Mass lesion shown by CT | | | | Diffuse injury°° (n 24) |
		Left nontemp (n 5)	Left temp (n 5)	Right (n 10)	Bilat (n 5)	
Storage	8/46	1/5	4/5	4/10	3/5	15/24
Consistent retrieval	7/46	—	5/5	4/10	3/5	16/24
Storage and/or retrieval	10/46	1/5	5/5	5/10	3/5	18/24

° A score was defined as defective if it fell at or below the 4th percentile of a same sex-subgroup of high school students (n 50). From Levin, H.S., and Eisenberg, H.M. Verbal learning and memory in relation to focal and diffuse effects of closed head injury. Presented at the Academy of Aphasia Meeting, 16 October 1979 in San Diego, California.

°° Denotes an injury producing coma without evidence of a mass lesion. Of 15 patients with diffuse injury who had CT, slit-like ventricles suggestive of swelling were seen in 11 cases.

with left temporal mass lesion than in patients with left hemisphere lesions confined to the frontal area or at least not primarily involving the temporal lobe ($p < 0.03$). Verbal long-term memory impairment, however, did not vary significantly between the left temporal group and patients with right hemisphere lesion (many of whom had long durations of coma).

The association between left temporal mass lesion and impairment of verbal memory and learning is in accord with previous findings of epileptic patients that show that left, but not right, temporal lobectomy disrupts verbal learning and memory (Milner, 1978; Weingartner, 1968). In contrast to the results obtained with epileptic patients who had seizure foci in their left hemisphere, the young closed head injury patients in our series had no evidence of previous neurologic dysfunction. Two of the five patients with left temporal mass lesion evidenced mild anomic disturbance at the time of testing, although three patients in the nontemporal group also exhibited mild language defect. The presence of measurable language deficit, which was characterized predominantly by anomic difficulty, was neither a necessary nor a sufficient condition for impaired learning and retention on the selective reminding test. Within the right hemisphere group, there was no patient with a mass lesion confined to the temporal lobe. Those patients with greater involvement of the temporal area generally performed no worse, or even better, than right hemisphere cases without temporal lobe involvement.

Persistence of verbal long-term memory deficit was assessed by serial selective reminding tests in 36 closed head injury patients (median age 20 years). Baseline evaluation was performed within six months of injury (median 39 days); the interval between the initial test and the followup assessment was at least six months. The median interval between the date of injury and the follow-up examination was one year. The series was comprised of ten mild injuries, seven patients with left hemisphere mass lesion (four were focal temporal), four with a right hemisphere lesion, three with bilateral mass lesion, and 12 with diffuse injuries. Despite the marked retrieval deficit found initially in all the patients with left temporal mass lesion, their followup scores were within normal limits. Of five patients with diffuse cerebral swelling shown by CT who were acutely impaired in retrieval, three recovered to within normal limits. Within the total series, 16 of the 22 patients with initial retrieval deficit had improved by the time of the followup test. Whereas the presence, or locus, of mass lesion was unrelated to long-term recovery, a Glasgow Coma Scale score of less than 8 at the time of hospitalization, evidence of acute oculovestibular deficit, persistent coma, and residual ventricular enlargement shown by serial CT scanning were correlates of persistent retrieval deficit. An exception to this pattern was a 44-year-old man (the oldest patient in the series) who evidenced residual retrieval deficit more than two years after sustaining an injury that produced compression of the left lateral ventricle, but no coma or neurologic deficit other than transient expressive aphasia.

In summary, disturbances of long-term storage and retrieval for verbal material are a frequent result of a closed head injury that produces mass lesion or diffuse injury. Focal involvement of the left temporal lobe and diffuse cerebral swelling suggested by CT findings are associated with early long-term memory impairment, whereas the severity of diffuse brain injury reflected by acute neurologic deficit, low scores on the Glasgow Coma Scale, and residual cerebral atrophy reflected by CT findings are related to persistent memory deficit.

Visual memory

Previous studies of patients with cerebral lesions other than closed head injury have established that damage to the right hemisphere frequently impairs visuospatial memory. Patients undergoing right temporal lobectomy for removal of epileptogenic tissue at the Montreal Neurologic Institute have been found to develop defective learning and retention of a block-tapping sequence (Milner, 1974), impaired continuous recognition memory (Kimura, 1963), and deficient recognition memory for photographs of faces (Milner, 1978). Posterior right hemisphere disease has been implicated in disturbed recognition memory for faces, particularly, but not exclusively, when a visual field defect is present (Warrington and James, 1967). In contrast, the Montreal studies have shown that left temporal lobectomy is relatively inconsequential with respect to visuospatial memory. Employing a continuous recognition memory task consisting of geometric designs interspersed with complex designs that were difficult to verbally encode, Kimura (1963) reported that right temporal lobectomy resulted in an excessive number of false alarm errors when patients were asked to distinguish between recurring designs and stimuli presented only once in the series.

On the basis of previous investigations of patients with focal brain disease and studies of the effects of temporal lobectomy, it might be anticipated that a mass lesion (e.g., hematoma) in the right hemisphere would result in a visual memory deficit, particularly if the lesion were situated in the temporal lobe or associated with a visual field defect. This prediction assumes that the effects of temporal lobectomy in epileptic patients correspond to sequelae of mass lesions in closed head injury. As described in the section on long-term memory, Levin and Eisenberg (1979c) found that the presence of left temporal mass lesion was related to verbal long-term memory impairment, at least within the first few months of recovery. Few studies of closed head injury, however, have employed appropriate tasks for detecting visual memory deficit; authors have not consistently analyzed the effects of mass lesion or even differentiated these patients from diffuse injuries. Comparison of visual memory for designs and the retention of verbal material is further complicated by variation in the retention interval and amount of information, both of which determine the level of difficulty.

E. Smith (1974) evaluated the presence of material-specific memory deficit at least ten years after closed head injury and, unexpectedly, found that patients with an impact to the right side of the head (as judged by the lines of fracture) were generally more impaired on both visuospatial and verbal tasks. Impact to the left frontal and right parietal areas was particularly likely to result in visual memory deficit. In the absence of direct evidence (e.g., CT scan, surgery) of lateralized brain damage, contused brain tissue adjacent to the site of impact and contrecoup effects are difficult to distinguish in this study.

Brooks (1972) studied visual memory after clearing of posttraumatic amnesia in 27 closed head injury patients by testing reproduction of geometric designs after each was presented for 10 sec, reproduction of the complex Rey design, and performance on the continuous recognition memory task of Kimura. The closed head injury group, which varied with respect to injury severity, performed below the level of an orthopedic control group on all tasks with the exception of reproduction of geometric designs. Duration of posttraumatic amnesia was related to the memory scores on all tasks, including such verbal tests as recall of paragraphs. Although Brooks reported that aphasic defect was unrelated to differential impairment on the geometric vs. complex designs of the recognition task, there was no description or analysis of focal mass lesions.

Recognition memory after closed head injury was further studied by Brooks (1974a) who administered Kimura's task to 34 patients after posttraumatic amnesia resolved (range of duration 2 to 300 days). In comparison with orthopedic patients, the closed head injury group had a lower corrected score (number of correct responses — number of false alarm errors of misidentifying a "new" stimulus as "old") and excessive false negative errors (i.e., stating that a previously presented old stimulus was "new"). The two groups did not differ, however, in the number of false alarm errors. The corrected total score and number of false alarms, but not false negative errors, correlated with posttraumatic amnesia duration; no measure of performance was related to the presence of neurologic signs. The scores of patients who were 30 years of age or older generally accounted for the correlation with posttraumatic amnesia. As in his previous study, Brooks approached the question of material-specific memory deficit by comparing the errors on geometric designs (easy to encode verbally)

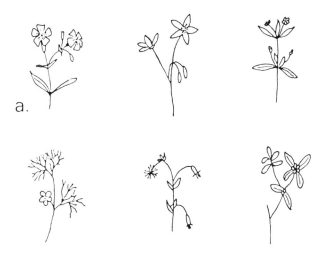

Fig. 5-6. An "old" stimulus (a) on the Continuous Recognition Memory Task and its five corresponding "new" stimuli.

and complex, amorphous designs (difficult to encode verbally) in aphasic patients who were assumed to have primarily left hemisphere damage as compared to nonaphasic patients. Although this analysis corroborated the previous finding (Brooks, 1972) that there is no relationship between the pattern of errors and aphasia, no radiologic or surgical documentation of lateralized mass lesion was reported. As noted in the section on language recovery, it is unusual, but still not very rare, for aphasic defects to occur in closed head-injured patients in whom focal neurologic deficit or CT findings suggest greater damage to the right hemisphere than the left hemisphere.

Continuous recognition memory after closed head injury was investigated by Hannay, Levin, and Grossman (1979), who used a series of 120 line drawings presented for 3 sec, each of which represented familiar categories of living things and objects (e.g., flowers, birds) as stimuli. Since the goal was to devise a task that would sustain the cooperation of even severely injured patients, the authors selected common environmental stimuli rather than unfamiliar visuospatial patterns that might have been frustrating for these patients. After the initial 20 trials in which all stimuli were "new," eight of these drawings reappeared in each of the following five trial blocks (20 trials each) and were thus "old" every time they were repeated. Of the 12 "new" stimuli in each trial block, eight represented one of the categories of recurring stimuli and four were from unrelated categories. Figure 5-6 depicts an old stimulus and five new stimuli perceptually similar to the old stimulus.

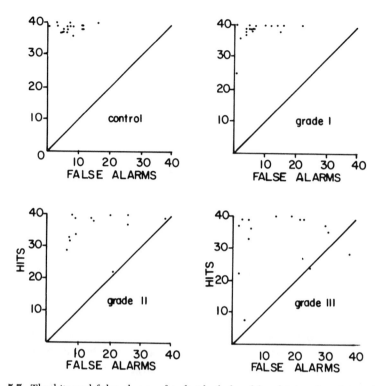

Fig. 5-7. The hits and false alarms of individual closed head-injured patients plotted separately for each injury group (I, no coma and normal neurologic findings; II, less than 24 hours of coma; III, greater than 24 hours of coma). [From Hannay, H.J. et al. (1979). Impaired recognition memory after head injury. *Cortex*, 15:269–283. Reproduced with permission of the authors and publisher.]

The patient was asked to state after each stimulus whether it was "old" or "new." As in Brooks' procedure, testing was deferred until posttraumatic amnesia resolved as measured by the GOAT. Severity of injury, as estimated by coma duration, was graded as I (no coma), II (0 to 24 hours), and III (over 24 hours); a control group of medical patients without evidence or history of brain damage was also studied. In contrast to the results reported by Brooks, Figure 5-7 shows that excessive false alarms (misidentifying a new stimulus as one previously seen) primarily differentiated the severe injuries from the mild closed head injury and control groups. Numerous false negative errors, i.e., misidentifying an old stimulus as new, were infrequent and generally confined to the most severe injuries. Duration of coma was correlated with the total number of correct responses, but not with either type of error taken individually. More than two-thirds of the cases with severe (II, III) closed head injury achieved a total score that fell below the range of scores in the control group. There was no relationship between educational level and any of the performance measures.

In a reanalysis of the data from the Hannay, Levin, and Grossman study, with additional cases of severe closed head injury, an attempt was made to determine whether the lateralization of mass lesions was related to continuous recognition memory. Dissociation of material-specific memory was confined to patients with left temporal mass lesions who exhibited normal continuous recognition memory on this task despite defective verbal learning and defective memory on the selective reminding task. Although only a few patients with right hemisphere mass lesion were given both tests, there was no corresponding dissociation of performance. The familiar, verbally codeable stimuli in the continuous recognition memory task might allow patients with visuospatial deficit to rely upon verbal processing, whereas patients with focal left hemisphere damage could employ a pattern recognition strategy on this task.

Signal detection analysis of memory

Impaired performance by head injured-patients on memory tasks is generally attributed to disturbance of at least one stage of memory, i.e., encoding, storage or retrieval. Conventional methods of testing memory do not preclude a shift in decision strategy or response criterion (e.g., a more cautious approach to stating that a stimulus was seen previously) as the basis for a decline in performance.

The signal detection theory of recognition memory (Lockhart and Murdock, 1970) postulates that the subject responds to two classes of stimuli, signal plus noise and noise alone. As depicted in Figure 5-8, noise is represented within the context of recognition memory by presentations of new items; signal plus noise trials correspond to old items. According to the theory, the distributions of sensory input from both noise and signal plus noise are assumed to be normal and to have a variance of 1. Signal detection theory assumes that the subject responds to these two types of trials that define separate probability density functions on the same axis (Figure 5-8) by determining whether the psychological effect of a given stimulus on this continuum exceeds some criterial value. From the proportions of hits and false alarms on the recognition memory task, a measure of sensitivity or mnemonic efficiency (d') is derived, which represents the difference between the means of the signal and signal plus noise distribu-

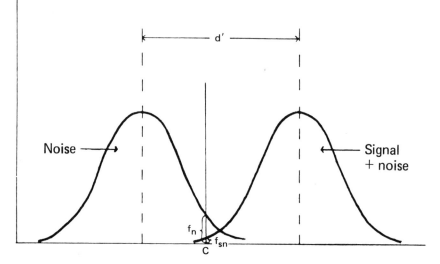

Amount of sensory input

Fig. 5-8. Probability density distributions of noise ("new") and signal plus noise ("old") denotes the value of sensory input above which the patient responds "old" and below which a "new" response is given. Efficient discrimination (high d' value) of old and new stimuli implies a greater separation of the noise and signal plus noise distributions (top), whereas deficient recognition memory implies overlapping noise and signal plus noise distribution (bottom of figure).

tions for a subject. To the degree that the distributions of sensory input produced by signal plus noise and noise overlap, the subject will be uncertain whether the sensory input derives from the presence of noise (new item) or a signal (old item). It is further assumed that the subject sets a response criterion (c) (Figure 5-8), a level of sensory input above which he responds that a signal (old item) was present and below which he states that the signal was absent (new item). Insofar as noise is assumed to be a normal variable with a variance of 1, it is possible to obtain a measure of c based on the probability of false alarms, i.e., $c = -Z[P(S/n)]$, where $P(S/n)$ is the probability of a false alarm. In early applications of signal detection theory to recognition memory, the parameter β was employed to assess response bias. It refers to the likelihood ratio, i.e., the ratio between the signal and signal plus noise density functions at the criterion (c).

Brooks (1974b) analyzed his continuous recognition memory data in terms of signal detection theory and found that closed head injury patients evidenced reduced memory efficiency as reflected by a lower d' value than the control group. He also reported a significantly higher response criterion (β) value, which led him to suggest that these patients were more cautious about identifying a stimulus as having been seen previously. Memory sensitivity, as measured by d', was inversely related to duration of posttraumatic amnesia, whereas no such relationship was obtained for β. Brooks' use of β as a measure of response criterion, which is held to be theoretically independent of d', has been criticized because it must then be assumed that the patient has an opportunity to estimate the values of the two probability distributions $P(s)$, $P(sn)$ and is capable of retaining this information across trials (Hannay et al., 1979; Richardson, 1979b). Given the relatively small number of trials used in a clinical study, the lack of feedback from the examiner, and the frequently impaired memory in closed head injury patients, the use of β as a measure of response bias in head-injured patients is inappropriate. Moreover, insofar as β is defined as the ratio of the ordinate of the signal plus noise distribution to the ordinate of the noise distribution at the subject's response criterion (c), β depends on the rate of hits as well as the rate of false alarms. Thus, β would be expected to vary inversely with memory sensitivity, i.e., patients with a low d' value would be likely to obtain high values of β.

Hannay, Levin and Grossman (1979) proposed that the response criterion c is a more appropriate measure because it is derived solely from the probability of false alarms. Richardson (1979b) reinterpreted Brooks's data in light of these considerations and concurred with the author that the memory sensitivity of the closed head injury patients was reduced, but he rejected the inference that the groups differed in terms of their criterion placement on the decision axis. Consistent with the results reported by Brooks, Hannay and her coworkers found that d' in patients with mild closed head injury exceeded the values obtained in grades II and III. The measure of response criterion c was lower for grade II patients (e.g., suggesting that they were less cautious in designating a drawing as old) as compared to the grade I (mild injury) and control groups. A similar trend for c in grade III patients only approached significance because of the greater variability in this group. Contrary to Brooks' suggestion that closed head injury patients might be more cautious in asserting that a stimulus had been seen previously, Hannay, Levin, and Grossman concluded that " . . . CHI sufficient to produce a memory deficit may result in patients setting a lower criterion for saying that they have seen the stimulus previously on this task." Memory sensitivity (d') and criterion (c) values were, however, frequently dissociated. Of the performance measures and signal detection indices only total correct responses and d' were significantly correlated with duration of coma.

Analysis of the efficiency of discrimination between the scores of closed head injury patients and the distribution of the scores of the control group disclosed that the values of d' and c in the head-injured patients more frequently fell outside the range of normal subjects as compared to the raw score measures of hits and false alarms.

In summary, application of signal detection theory to recognition memory holds considerable promise both as a research technique and as an index to characterize recovery. The format of continuous recognition memory lends itself to multiple forms that could be given serially to determine changes in d' values. The practical advantages include the minimal demands posed by recognition memory on verbal or motor responses and its suitability for bedside examination.

6. Cognitive effects

Intellectual recovery

Intellectual recovery after head injury has profound implications for vocational rehabilitation, adjustment to the activities of daily living, and social reintegration. As will be seen in the studies discussed below, cognitive impairment of greater or lesser degree is shown by many patients with closed head injury or penetrating brain wounds. Moreover, recent improvements in emergency patient transport and neurosurgical treatment of acute closed head injury (Becker et al., 1977), which reduce preventable mortality (e.g., secondary brain damage resulting from hypoxia), no doubt will result in a larger number of survivors with significant cognitive defects. It appears that, despite early definitive treatment, posttraumatic dementia is particularly likely to occur in cases of brain injury of the immediate impact type in which massive shearing of axons occurs at the moment of trauma (cf. Adams et al., 1977).

Considering the major implications of intellectual deficit for postinjury functioning, relatively few studies dealing with this question have been reported. Methodological deficiencies, which are found to a varying degree in the studies summarized in Table 6-1 of cognition after head injury, include (1) lack of information concerning preinjury cognitive ability; (2) the absence of an appropriate control group, when indicated; (3) failure to screen for preinjury conditions (e.g., alcoholism) that potentially compromise cognitive efficiency; (4) inadequate documentation of acute closed head injury severity that often obscures neurologic heterogeneity; and (5) lack of control of the injury-test interval and lack of serial testing to depict the time-course of recovery. These shortcomings impose constraints on generalizing from any single published study of intellectual recovery after closed head injury.

Table 6-1. Intellectual recovery after closed head injury[a]

Author/country	Selection criteria	Age at injury	Injury/test interval	Preinjury information/control group	Cognitive measures	Overall results	Neurologic indices investigated
Becker (1975) USA	Enlisted men with CHI (n 10); no other criteria stated	$\bar{x} = 20$	Subacute post-PTA; retest 10–11 wks after injury	Est $\bar{x}$ IQ = 107 from GCT scores; control group matched to this est IQ using WAIS	WAIS given twice to CHI and control group	CHI patients improved esp on Block Design & Digit Span, but below the matched controls. $\bar{x}$ Verb IQ = 101, $\bar{x}$ Perf IQ = 96 on retest. Improvement over 11-week interval in both groups	None
Benayoun et al. (1969) France	All patients had coma or PTA (n 28)	15–42 ($\bar{x}$ not stated)	$\bar{x} = 15$ d after coma	Normal control group—matching was unspecified	WAIS	59% CHI cases had Verb IQ < 85; 70% < 85 on Perf; 15% controls had < 85 on Verb, Perf; increased "scatter" in CHI	None
Black (1973) USA	Servicemen with CHI (n 50) vs. penetrating missile (n 50); no other criteria stated	$\bar{x} = 22$	$\bar{x} = 3$ mos	$\bar{x}$ educ 11 yrs in CHI vs. 12 yrs in penetrating	WAIS, Shipley-Hartford	$\bar{x}$ Full Scale IQ = 96 (penetrating) vs. 85 (CHI); Shipley $\bar{x}$ IQ = 93 (penetrating) vs. 79 (CHI)	None
Dencker (1960), Dencker & Lofving (1958) Sweden	MZ twins discordant for CHI (30 pairs, 28 tested); no "intracranial complications"	10–60	$\bar{x} = 10$ yrs (3–25)	MZ co-twins	Raven's Matrices, Abstraction, Digit Span	CHI probands had worse scores on abstraction, but not Raven's	Probands with PTA > 10 min did not differ in outcome from cases with briefer PTA

Study	Age	Sample	Follow-up/PTA	Test	Education/Control	Results	Correlates
Gronwall (1976b, 1977); Gronwall & Sampson (1974); Gronwall & Wrightson (1974) New Zealand	17–25 yrs	Consecutive CHI, no hematoma, skull fx, or previous injury (n 80); "post-concussion Sx" (n 10). Control CHI (matched to post-concussional, n 10). Mild (PTA < 24 hr) & moderate (PTA 1–7 d) injuries	5–35 d ("post-concussion"); < 48 hrs (control) consecutive cases	PASAT given serially until performance was normal	Approx. 3 yrs of secondary school in CHI and non-CHI groups	CHI patients recover on PASAT ≤ 35 d; recovery is prolonged in cases with post-concussional Sx; PASAT curve parallels readiness for return to work	PASAT performance positively related to PTA duration
Klwe & Cleeland (1972) USA	16–42	CHI patients referred to testing (n 100); excluded cases with previous injury	≤ 24 mos	Halstead-Reitan, including WAIS	None; used normative data for comparison	Perf IQ was more strongly related to neurologic indices than was Verb IQ. Showed intercorrelation among neurologic variables	Perf IQ differentiated patients who had post neurologic findings, hematoma, and longer coma (when tested ≥ 7 mos postinjury); Categories reflected coma duration.** Skull fx unrelated to cognitive recovery
Levin et al. (1979) USA	Mdn = 21	Glasgow Coma Scale score ≤ 8, age 16–50 (n 27), exclusion of cases with previous CHI, ETOH, or drug abuse. Glasgow Outcome Scale used to stratify patients	≥ 6 mos, Mdn = 12 mos	WAIS	Mdn educ = 12; no significant difference in education according to outcome (e.g. Good Recovery vs. Severe Disability)	Mdn overall Verb IQ = 93, Perf IQ = 90; IQ in severely disabled patients (Verb IQ = 66, Perf IQ = 60) was significantly below that of Good Recovery (Verb IQ = 94, Perf IQ = 100) and Moderate Disability (Verb IQ = 90, Perf IQ = 90). Moderately disabled patients were below that of cases with Good Recovery	Acute aphasia related to lower Verb IQ at followup; acute hemiparesis and nonreactive pupils related to Perf IQ; occulovestibular deficit was predictive of low Verb & Perf IQ

Table 6-1. Intellectual recovery after closed head injury° (continued)

Author/country	Selection criteria	Age at injury	Injury/test interval	Preinjury information/control group	Cognitive measures	Overall results	Neurologic indices investigated
Mandleberg (1975) UK	n_1 16 CHI cases in PTA ($\bar{x}$ = 110 d) n_2 16 CHIs out of PTA ($\bar{x}$ = 19 d)	$\bar{x}$ = 20	On initial test (2 mos) group 1 in PTA, group 2 out of PTA; followup at 18, 20 mos	$\bar{x}$ educ = 10 yrs	WAIS	Group 1 < Group 2 especially on Perf IQ (51 vs 80), but also on Verb IQ (75 vs 99); no differences on followup	Motor deficit, aphasia & hematoma related to initial scores; only aphasia and hematoma related to followup IQ
Mandleberg (1976) UK	n 51; $\bar{x}$ PTA = 6 wks, 4 subgroups based on PTA; n 98 in replication; $\bar{x}$ PTA = 5 wks	$\bar{x}$ = 29; x = 35 in study 2	Serial—3, 6, 12, 30 mos	None given; study compared CHI subgroups	WAIS	PTA duration related to Verb IQ at 3 mos, but not later; PTA duration related to Perf IQ at 6 & 9 mos, but not later; in long-term, PTA duration not prognostic of IQ	PTA duration found to be predictive of IQ scores only up to 6–9 mos
Mandleberg & Brooks (1975) UK	n = 40 CHI, PTA > 4 d	$\bar{x}$ = 28	Serial—3, 5, 10, 36 mos	$\bar{x}$ educ = 10 yrs; control group-psych patients, $\bar{x}$ age = 32 yrs, $\bar{x}$ educ = 10 yrs	WAIS	Verb IQ improved up to 5 mos; Perf IQ improved up to 13 mos; at 36 mos, CHI patients' IQs were similar to controls	None

Study	Subjects	Age	Interval	Control/Education	Tests	Results	Conclusions
Norrman & Savahn (1961) Sweden	CHI with coma > 1 wk (n 28)	16->49	2 yrs	$\bar{x}$ educ = grade school; matched control group (neurotics)	Kohs Blocks; synonyms	CHI < controls on Kohs Blocks, but not different on synonyms	Block construction was the only test related to PTA
Roberts (1980) UK	Consecutive admissions with PTA ≥ 1 wk—subgroup tested (n 77); excluded women, left-handers, cases requiring intracranial surgery for hematomas, patients with depressed fx, patients whose ability to complete the tests was uncertain	5–85	10–24 yrs	Not specifically cited; no control group	Raven's Progressive Matrices, Mill Hill Vocab, WAIS Block Design, & Maze Test	Long PTA (≥ 5 wks) cases had lower Raven's scores than short PTA patients; impact to right parietal area was associated with defective block construction	Side and locus of impact related to WAIS Block Designs & maze performance in the case of right parietal patients. Visuospatial ability was affected more by PTA duration than was verbal ability

Table 6-1. Intellectual recovery after closed head injury° (continued)

Author/country	Selection criteria	Age at injury	Injury/test interval	Preinjury information/control group	Cognitive measures	Overall results	Neurologic indices investigated
Ruesch (1946) USA	(a) Consecutive admissions for CHI examined (n 70); serially tested 53 (b) CHIs tested ≤ 48 hrs (n_1 40) vs. CHI unable to be tested as soon because of coma or confusion (n_2 50) (c) CHI with hematoma or fx (n 15) vs. "uncomplicated" cases (n 33)	(a) $\bar{x}$ = 39 (b) $\bar{x}_1$ = 40 $\bar{x}_2$ = 36 (c) NA	(a) ≤ 24 hrs, retest during hospitalization, 4–12 wks in cases serially tested (b) < 48 hrs or later (c) 5.53 d	$\bar{x}$ educ = 8 yrs, all groups	(a,b) Serial 7s, visuomotor task, Wechsler-Bellevue Comprehension, Coding, Similarities, Picture Discrim, Digit Span, & Block Designs, (c) Special tests—color naming speed	(a) Serial scores showed the series (n 53) could be divided into 2 groups, improved (n 28) vs nonimproved (n 25) by 4–12 wks. On first test, 7s was failed most often (61%); on last test visuomotor test was most sensitive (60%); verbal comprehension was most resistant. For 70 CHIs tested 1–3 mos, Full Scale (prorated) IQ = 95; Verb Perf disparity not present (b) Naming speed was initially impaired in 50% of series & recovered in all cases	(a) Patients with deficit on last test had longer coma & confusion than cases who improved. At 1–3 mos, 17 cases with fx or subdural hematoma did not differ from CHI with coma only (n 53). Intellectual impairment at 3 mos was found only in cases with confusion ≥ 19 d after injury (b) CHIs who could not be tested ≤ 48 hrs had more complications (e.g. fx, bloody spinal fluid (c) "Complicated" CHIs performed similarly to cases with coma without complications on naming speed and other special tests given at 53 d

Study	Sample	$\bar{x}$	Time tested	ETOH/history	Test	IQ results	Comments
Ruesch & Bowman (1945) (USA)	"Chronic" CHIs tested ≥ 3 mos with signs of brain damage (n_1 58); "chronic" without signs (n_2 67); acute CHI (n_3 47)	$\bar{x}_1 = 33$ $\bar{x}_2 = 38$ $\bar{x}_3 = 47$	≥ 3 mos in chronic, ≤ 4 wks in acute	ETOH abuse in history of % of chronic & % of acute cases; % of chronics had previous CHI. Control group (neurotics) (n 40) $\bar{x}$ age = 34. Educ not given	Wechsler Bellevue	$\bar{x}$ Full Scale IQ 96 in acute, 101 in chronics with signs, 108 in chronics, without signs, & 109 in controls	Signs of brain damage included persistent confusion, cranial nerve findings, seizures, bloody spinal fluid, or pathologic reflexes
Ruesch & Moore (1943) USA	Consecutive admissions (n 190)	$\bar{x} = 29$	≤ 24 hrs	NA	Serial 7s, Digit Span, other brief tests	64% of patients could be tested. Serial 7s was the most sensitive test	Indices most related to incapacity to take tests and impaired scores were bloody spinal fluid & ETOH history
Uzzell et al. (1979) USA	CHI with initial and follow-up CT scans who were oriented when tested; left mass lesion (n_1 8), right lesion (n_2 13), diffuse bilateral (n_3 5)	$\bar{x}_1 = 29$ $\bar{x}_2 = 31$ $\bar{x}_3 = 37$	Within 6 mos except for 2 cases tested at 7–11 mos	$\bar{x}$ educ = 10, 12 and 11 years, respectively. Pertinent pre-CHI history not given	WAIS	$\bar{x}$ Verb IQ = 72, $\bar{x}$ Perf IQ = 81 for left lesion; $\bar{x}$ Verb IQ = 96; $\bar{x}$ Perf IQ = 79 for right lesion; $\bar{x}$ Verb IQ = 87, $\bar{x}$ Perf IQ = 77 for diffuse bilateral	The groups with lateralized mass lesions differed most consistently on the Verb subtests and on Digit Symbol and Picture Arrangement subtests of Perf Scale
Vigouroux et al. (1972) France	CHIs selected because of suspected dementia (n 51)	Mostly young adults	1–10 yrs	NA	WAIS	$\bar{x}$ Verb IQ = 96, $\bar{x}$ Perf IQ = 90; 39% had Verb IQ ≥ 100 vs. 24% for Perf IQ	Ventricular enlargement was frequently present but not studied in relation to cognition

Abbreviations: CHI, closed head injury; d, days; est, estimated; ETOH, alcohol; fx, fracture; GCT, General Classification Test; hr, hour; mdn, median; mos, months; MZ, monozygotic; n, number; NA, not available; PASAT, Paced Auditory Serial Addition Test; Perf, performance; posit, positive; psych, psychiatric; PTA, posttraumatic amnesia; sx, symptoms; Verb, Verbal; WAIS, Wechsler Adult Intelligence Test; wk, week; $\bar{x}$, mean; yr, year.

*Studies that include penetrating missile wounds were not considered; neuropsychologic variables other than intellectual ability and information processing rate are reviewed in other chapters.

**Categories Test evaluates abstract problem solving and shifting of response set across trials.

Ascertainment of preinjury level

In a study of intellectual deficit subsequent to penetrating missile wounds of the brain in soldiers, Weinstein and Teuber (1957) compared the scores on the Army General Classification Test at the time of military induction to the results at the time of long-term followup. In civilian head injury, military and school records are the only source of information to estimate preinjury ability. General Classification Test scores and group administered standardized tests in schools may be interpreted as approximations of the IQ level obtained in an individual examination (e.g., WAIS). Serial test scores found in high school records, which show stability in percentile rank, aid considerably in estimating the degree of postinjury deficit in a young adult. In the absence of preinjury test data, investigators have employed various strategies to evaluate the degree of cognitive recovery.

Becker (1975) obtained the General Classification Test scores at the time of military induction for young servicemen who subsequently sustained closed head injury. However, in contrast to the Weinstein and Teuber approach of employing the General Classification Test as an outcome measure, Becker used the information to select a control group whose Wechsler IQs approximated the preinjury classification scores of the head-injured patients. He also retested the control group on the WAIS at an interval to coincide with the followup assessment of the head-injured cases. School records were reported by Norrman and Svahn (1961), but were not used to measure recovery. From regression studies of IQ based on educational level, Ruesch and his coworkers concluded that consecutively admitted closed head injury patients were from one-half to one standard deviation below average when tested within three months after injury. Dencker and Löfring (1958) utilized the concordance in IQ between monozygotic twins by selecting for long-term followup twin pairs in which the proband had sustained a closed head injury. In the absence of any premorbid estimate of intellectual level, Mandleberg and Brooks (1975) included a control group matched to closed head injury patients for educational level. Intellectual recovery was thereby inferred when the serial WAIS scores of the head-injured patients reached the level of the control group. Inclusion of psychiatric patients (including alcoholics) in the control group may have reduced the possibility of discovering a deficit in the head-injured patients.

In an ongoing study of long-term cognitive outcome, Levin (1981) compared the recovery of patients after severe closed head injury to findings obtained in patients with similar demographic background who had sustained only mild injury with no evidence of neurologic deficit, loss of consciousness of more than a few minutes duration, or abnormal CT scan when it was performed. Similarly, Levin, Grossman, Rose, and Teasdale (1979) compared intellectual recovery in subgroups of head-injured patients who were divided, for statistical purposes, according to the presence of acute neurologic deficit (e.g., oculovestibular findings) and were otherwise comparable with respect to educational and socioeconomic background. Any systematic difference in cognitive level at the time of followup can be reasonably attributed to the variation in the severity of brain injury. This research strategy is facilitated by restricting the range of preinjury heterogeneity, i.e., excluding patients with potential intellectual defects arising from early neurologic insult, alcoholism, or neuropsychiatric disorder.

Selection criteria

Comparisons of cognitive recovery across different series of patients would be facilitated by standardization of criteria in the selection of patients for study. A uniform procedure in screening for preinjury conditions that are potentially related to intellectual deficit would clarify the interpretation of differences in cognitive outcome. Whether participation in an outcome study is open to consecutively admitted head injuries or restricted to patients on the basis of neurologic findings (e.g., a minimum coma scale score or duration of posttraumatic amnesia) is also a major factor to be considered in selection. Table 6-1 includes the selection criteria employed in studies of cognitive recovery. Although it is to be expected that the presence and lateralization of mass effect differentially impair verbal and visuospatial abilities, it is apparent from Table 6-1 that many studies have not reported the presence of hematoma or have not analyzed the data of these patients separately. Analyzing the effects of hematoma per se without regard to its cerebral localization may obscure its effects on cognition.

It is also apparent from Table 6-1 that most studies have failed to screen for (or at least report) preinjury conditions that could have altered preinjury cognitive efficiency and possibly interacted with the effects of closed head injury. In view of the demographic profiles of patients at risk for head injury (Field, 1976) it is regrettable that the findings on alcoholics usually have not been segregated from those on other patients. The protocol followed by Levin and his coworkers (1979) excluded patients who were alcoholics or chronic drug abusers from the study of cognitive outcome on the ground that there is no information available that can be used to differentiate the contributions of these conditions from the effects of head injury with respect to cognitive sequelae.

Neurologic indices of acute injury

Inspection of Table 6-1 indicates that only a few studies have characterized the severity of acute injury beyond estimating the duration of posttraumatic amnesia. Furthermore, there exist no widely accepted criteria or quantitative scales for its assessment. In several instances (cf. Mandleberg and Brooks, 1975), it has been estimated retrospectively by questioning the patients at the time of long-term followup. Excessive measurement error in assessing posttraumatic amnesia may account for its reported relatively low relationship to cognitive outcome after six to nine months postinjury (Mandleberg, 1976).

Since the early studies by Ruesch and his colleagues in which injury complications such as hematoma were analyzed, only a few investigators have evaluated the effects indicated by neurologic indices (e.g., Kløve and Cleeland, 1972; Levin et al., 1979; Mandleberg, 1975). A recent brief report by Uzzell, Zimmerman, Dolinskas, and Obrist (1979) showed that early CT findings may differentiate closed head injury patients with respect to different cognitive sequelae. In a study of long-term cognitive outcome, Levin, Grossman, Rose, and Teasdale (1979) accepted the serial neurologic findings for analysis only after detailed review by three neurosurgeons. If it may be assumed that variables related to survival and global functioning after severe closed head injury are relevant to cognitive recovery, it is clear that future studies should consider serial scores on a quantitative coma scale, neurologic findings, and CT scan results in the documentation of head injury severity.

Injury-test interval

Variation across studies with respect to the interval between the dates of injury and intellectual assessment is depicted in Table 6-1. The time course of these studies may be classified as (1) subacute, i.e., evaluation during the first two days after mild closed head injury (cf. Gronwall and Sampson, 1974; Ruesch and Moore, 1943) or shortly after resolution of posttraumatic amnesia (cf. Becker, 1975); (2) long-term ($\geq$ six months) follow-up, generally of severe closed head injury (cf. Roberts, 1979); and (3) serial follow-up with multiple testing of each patient (cf. Mandleberg and Brooks, 1975).

Physicians and families of patients frequently ask the psychologist to estimate the minimum interval sufficient to observe the full extent of intellectual recovery. Vocational planning by rehabilitation specialists and the development of realistic expectations by the patient's family are influenced by prognostic information bearing on the estimated period of mental recovery.

Integration of the findings summarized in Table 6-1 leads to the conclusion that the briefest interval sufficient to measure the peak level of recovery varies according to the severity of injury. In a study of patients with apparently mild closed head injury, Becker (1975) found substantial recovery on the WAIS over an 11-week period.

Determination of the minimum time period sufficient to measure the full extent of intellectual recovery is more complicated in severe closed head injury. As shown in Table 6-1, the Glasgow studies included serial WAIS administration over the course of approximately three years. These investigators concluded that after severe closed head injury (posttraumatic amnesia over one week), the recovery curve for Verbal IQ usually reaches a plateau by six to 12 months, whereas increments in Performance IQ may continue for a year or more after injury. Notwithstanding the guidelines suggested by the Glasgow studies, there is considerable individual variation in rate of recovery after severe closed head injury reflecting such factors as preinjury ability, and age, and the presence of focal mass lesion and other neurologic findings (Benton, 1979b; Levin et al., 1979). It is also possible that handedness and, by inference, the pattern of cerebral dominance may affect the recovery of Verbal IQ. Serial examination of patient subgroups classified by acute neurologic and CT findings and demographic variables would further elucidate the time-course for restitution of function.

Cognitive measures and practice effects

Review of the studies in Table 6-1 leads to the formulation that early administration of brief measures of cognitive speed (e.g., serial 7s, the PASAT test of Gronwall) yields clinically useful recovery curves in mildly injured patients. As is evident from the table, there is a preference among investigators for employing the WAIS as a cognitive outcome measure, particularly for the determination of long-term recovery after severe closed head injury. In contrast to alternative tests (e.g., Raven's Progressive Matrices), the WAIS permits a direct comparison of different abilities and yields a profile of subtest scores. Interpretation of the WAIS scores is facilitated by the availability of comprehensive standardization data for a wide distribution of ages. Direct comparison of Wechsler IQ results in children (WISC-R) to those obtained in adults facilitates the investigation of "plasticity" after closed head injury.

Objections to serial examination by the WAIS include potential practice effects because the test lacks parallel forms. Concern about the effects of repeated exposure to test materials applies primarily to such Performance Scale subtests as Object Assembly, in which the solution of puzzles may be remembered. In a comparison of patients with mild closed head injury and a control group matched on estimated preinjury IQ, Becker (1975) reported substantial improvement in both groups upon retesting after 10 weeks. Differential increments between the groups varied with the WAIS subtest; head-injured patients, but not control subjects, showed significant gains on the Digit Span and Block Design subtests, whereas the increment in the noninjured group was greater on other subtests, particularly Object Assembly, Picture Completion, and Comprehension. Serial study of severe closed head injury patients with wider spacing of test administrations was undertaken by Mandleberg and Brooks (1975), who compared the three-year followup scores of patients differing in the number of times (one through four) the WAIS had been given to them. They found no evidence for practice effects insofar as the three-year WAIS scores were not related to the number of previous testings. This finding is congruent with our own observation that severely injured patients, evaluated at six- to 12-month intervals, frequently deny having previously seen the test materials. In summary, multiple administrations of the WAIS over a period of several months probably produce significant practice effects in patients with relatively mild injury, but not in severely injured patients who are serially tested at widely separated intervals.

Intellectual recovery: A synthesis of previous studies

After considering the aforementioned methodologic problems and variation in procedure across studies, one may be reluctant to accept any integration of their findings. Although caution in drawing conclusions is justified, it is encouraging that most studies of long-term intellectual recovery have employed the WAIS. This degree of standardization in cognitive measurement is appreciated when one considers the vast procedural differences in studies evaluating functions such as memory, language, and perception after head injury.

Early intellectual recovery

Systematic study of cognitive functioning during the early stages of recovery from closed head injury was launched in the 1940s by Ruesch and his coworkers (Table 6-1), who reported their findings for consecutive head injury admissions to the Boston City Hospital. Although the investigation of consecutive cases produced a series that was heterogeneous with respect to the severity of injury, the authors attempted to differentiate the effects of various neurologic indices in their analysis of the data. They also supplemented the subtests of the Wechsler-Bellevue Scale (the predecessor of the WAIS) with measures of cognitive speed (serial 7s, naming speed), visuomotor speed, fatigability, and perception. They found that patients with brief periods of coma and/or confusion and no hematoma recovered markedly on these measures within one to three months of injury (Table 6-1).

In a series of studies of groups of closed head injury patients who were fairly homogeneous with respect to injury severity and antecedent neuropsychiatric history, Gronwall and her colleagues have elucidated the early slowing of information processing rate and the time-course of its recovery. They challenged the cognitive capacity of closed head injury patients and control groups by varying the rate of stimulus presentation on a task of simple addition, i.e., the Paced Auditory Serial Addition Test (PASAT). Gronwall's PASAT involves the tape-recorded presentation of a random series of digits (1 through 9) to the patient who is instructed to add pairs of numbers such that each number is added to the one immediately preceding it. For example, if the first three numbers are 1, 4, and 7, the patient's response would be 5 after the second digit is presented and 11 after the third digit is presented. The patient is asked to respond verbally before presentation of the next number. This test requires auditory processing of each item, holding the item in short-term memory for addition to the next digit and performing at a pace that corresponds to the interstimulus interval. Unpaced and paced practice trials are given to ensure comprehension of instructions and correct addition. Figure 6-1 indicates that the level of performance declines as the interval between digits is reduced. Gronwall initially tested mostly mild closed head injury patients within 48 hours of admission if they could respond verbally. The test was repeated every 24 hours until the patient was discharged (about one to five days after admission).

Figure 6-1 depicts initial impairment in the "severe concussion" (posttraumatic amnesia of one hour to seven days) group; despite considerable improvement on the final retest given four weeks after discharge, the patient's performances were far below that of the mild concussion and control groups. Mildly concussed patients (posttraumatic amnesia under one hour) differed from the control group on the initial test but the gap in performance was closed by the time of followup. Gronwall and Wrightson (1974) found that nearly all patients admitted to the hospital for mild closed head injury (posttraumatic amnesia under 24 hours) attained a normal rate of information processing on the PASAT by 35 days after injury. Followup assessment (one to three years postinjury) in an air pressure chamber simulating a high altitude condition has demonstrated

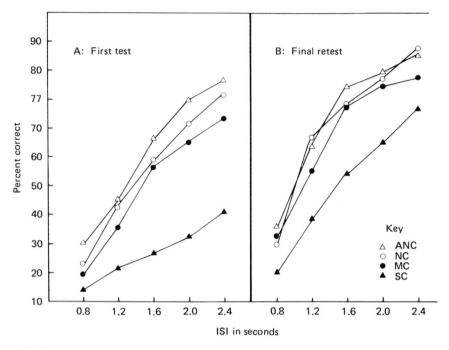

Fig. 6-1. Mean percentage correct PASAT as function of interstimulus interval on first test and final retest. (From Gronwall, D.M., and Sampson, H. (1974). *The Psychological Effects of Concussion.* Auckland University Press. Reproduced with permission of the authors and publisher.)

that a "latent" deficit on the PASAT can persist after minor closed head injury (Ewing, McCarthy, Gronwall, and Wrightson, 1980).

In a more recent serial study of early recovery from closed head injury in university students and less educated, but otherwise closely matched head-injured patients, Gronwall (1976b) reported that the time-course of recovery and the asymptotic level of performance on the PASAT were comparable. In contrast to similarly depressed levels of vocabulary and verbal fluency in the two groups shortly after hospital admission, the followup evaluation disclosed higher scores on these measures in the university students. Although replication of this study based on a small series (12 patients in a group) is warranted before drawing conclusions, the results suggest the possibility that the PASAT may be given without correction for differences in educational attainment.

From these observations, it is clear that impairment of cognitive processing in closed head injury patients becomes increasingly evident as the time for presentation of information is compressed. Under untimed conditions, such patients may perform satisfactorily. Insofar as Gronwall found that recovery on the PASAT was correlated with fitness for work, it appears that a "cognitive stress test" such as the PASAT might well be included in neuropsychological assessment after head injury. This procedure would seem to be particularly useful in evaluating return to occupations that involve sustained attention and rapid decision-making. However, completion of the PASAT during the initial hospitalization may exceed the ability of severe closed head injury patients to cooperate.

Long-term intellectual recovery

Intellectual recovery data are more abundant for long-term and serial studies of closed head injury than for the early phases of recovery. The findings in Table 6-1 indicate that there is substantial disagreement in the literature concerning the potential for restitution of intellectual functioning. Advocates of the view that intellectual ability eventually recovers to the normal level after closed head injury often have cited Dencker's study of monozygotic twin pairs in which the probands sustained a closed head injury. Dencker (1960) administered a series of tests to the twin pairs at least three years after injury and found that a test of abstraction was the only measure that differentiated the head-injured proband. "Severe" closed head injury, however, was defined as producing a posttraumatic amnesia of over ten minutes. Consequently, it is not surprising that a very limited effect of injury severity on subsequent cognitive function was found. In view of the scant description of acute injury severity provided by Dencker, it is difficult to reconcile his results with those of other studies.

Serial findings in the Glasgow studies have shown that WAIS IQ scores, which were consistently impaired during posttraumatic amnesia, eventually reached a plateau at the average level for adults (about six months for Verbal IQ, about 13 months for Performance IQ) and did not differ from those of a control group. Mandleberg and Brooks (1975) inferred that "it may be said that the cognitive abilities of the head injured patients *as a group* eventually returned to normal levels, despite the severity of their injuries as assessed by duration of PTA." The authors interpreted their findings as compatible with the conclusions reached earlier by Dencker. A more cautious interpretation of the Glasgow findings is that recovery of intelligence to within the average range (90 to 110 IQ) is common after a closed head injury that has produced a posttraumatic amnesia of at least one week. As noted earlier, the control group studied by Mandleberg and

Brooks included alcoholics and psychiatric patients, which might have led to an underestimate of the preinjury functioning of head injury cases. In the absence of an estimate of preinjury IQ, it is tenuous to presume recovery to a "normal level," particularly on a test known to measure marked individual differences in ability. That posttraumatic amnesia was predictive of IQ only up to nine months after injury may reflect the effects of other neurologic indices and error in measuring duration of amnesia.

Employing selection criteria (posttraumatic amnesia over one week) similar to the Glasgow studies, Norrman and Svahn (1961) found that amnesia duration was related to performance on the Kohs Block Designs (similar to those used in the WAIS) two years after injury. This finding was confirmed by Roberts (1979), who reported that intellectual deficit (WAIS subtests) at least ten years after injury was associated with a posttraumatic amnesia duration exceeding five weeks. Consistent with the possibility that the duration of impaired consciousness may have long-range implications for cognition, Kløve and Cleeland (1972) found that variation in the period of coma was reflected in the Performance Scale IQ when patients were tested at least seven months after injury, but not when they were evaluated earlier.

The prognostic significance of acute neurologic deficit other than posttraumatic amnesia or coma duration has been established. The Glasgow studies showed that early recovery (two months) was adversely affected by the presence of acute motor deficit, aphasia, and hematoma, whereas only the latter two indices were related to WAIS scores at 20 months after injury. In support of these results, other investigators (Kløve and Cleeland, 1972; Levin et al., 1979) documented the far-reaching consequences of acute neurologic deficit (Table 6-1). Levin, Grossman, Rose, and Teasdale (1979) were unable to substantiate the effects of intracranial hematoma, but their negative findings in a small series of patients must be interpreted cautiously. In contrast, Uzzell, Zimmerman, Dolinskas, and Obrist (1979) found differential effects on the Verbal IQ or Performance IQ according to the lateralization of intracranial hematoma or hemorrhagic contusion by CT. The authors reported that patients with right hemisphere mass lesions had a Verbal IQ above that of the group with left hemisphere lesions, but the groups did not differ significantly in Performance IQ. The effects of a mass lesion combined with diffuse cerebral swelling may produce devastating intellectual impairment.

Statistical arguments can be invoked against the approach of correlating acute neurologic findings with subsequent intellectual ability because neurologic indices can frequently be correlated with each other. This circumstance invites spurious correlations between cognitive recovery and neurologic variables. After noting that oculovestibular disturbance was related to both prolonged coma and profound cognitive deficit, Levin and his coworkers matched seven index cases to closed head injury patients with comparable coma duration who exhibited normal oculovestibular functioning. Long-term Performance IQ was impaired in both groups (median of 74 vs. 77), whereas Verbal IQ was clearly superior in patients who were spared oculovestibular deficit (100 vs. 73, $p < 0.05$). In a larger series of patients, multiple discriminant analysis could be utilized to examine the effects of various acute neurologic deficits, to adjust for their intercorrelations, and to derive an index of their specific contributions to predicting cognitive outcome.

This section began with a statement endorsing the assessment of intellectual recovery after closed head injury because of the anticipated relationship between the findings and the overall social and vocational adjustment in these patients. Ecologic validity of the WAIS with respect to global quality of adjustment in the community was supported by our finding that ratings on the Glasgow Outcome Scale correspond to the WAIS IQ (Levin et al., 1979). As summarized in Table 6-1, the Performance IQ was particularly relevant to overall outcome and was essentially independent of educational background (Spearman Rank Difference Correlation Coefficient, 0.10). Severe disability was uniformly associated with marked cognitive impairment. In contrast, patients who had attained a good recovery (nine out of ten returned to full time gainful employment) consistently scored within one standard deviation of the population mean on the WAIS, and several were above average. These patients emerged from relatively brief coma (median 24 hours before responding to commands) and had normal pupillary and oculovestibular findings on serial neurologic examination, despite an initial Glasgow Coma Scale score of 8 or less at the time of admission.

What can be expected of long-term cognitive functioning a year or two after injury? Providing that there is evidence to document, or at least suggest, normal preinjury intelligence, the encouraging recovery curves of the Glasgow studies portray a reasonably accurate prognosis for patients with only moderate coma duration (perhaps one to three days) uncomplicated by oculovestibular deficit or nonreactive pupils, which are often regarded as signs of brain stem injury. Given an at least average level of premorbid intelligence, greater confidence can be given to the prediction of recovery to an at least low average (IQ $\geq$ 90) range of intelligence if the patient was also spared an intracranial hematoma, hemiparesis, and aphasia. Although the findings to date suggest that the role of these factors is minor in comparison with oculovestibular and pupillary functioning, a firm basis for statistical prediction awaits further study.

7. Language functions

Aphasia is probably the earliest recorded neuropsychologic sequel of head injury. The Papyrus Ebers (Ebbel, 1937) indicates that Egyptian surgeons were familiar with posttraumatic speechlessness. Valerius Maximus (*ca.* A.D. 30) described a learned man of Athens who showed a specific impairment of memory for letters after being struck in the head by a stone (Benton and Joynt, 1960). This may be the earliest reference to traumatic alexia in Western literature.

Until recently, the study of posttraumatic aphasia consisted largely of investigations of patients who had sustained penetrating missile wounds of the brain in military action (cf. Russell and Espir, 1961). These injuries are typically produced by small metal fragments of high explosive shells that enter the brain from the point of impact and produce circumscribed brain injury in some cases. That missile injury can produce a restricted area of lesion is suggested by the finding of severe aphasia concomitant with focal motor deficit and minimal or no alteration of consciousness. As a consequence, the classical types of aphasia are more commonly observed in patients with missile wounds of the brain than in cases of blunt head trauma.

From the report of Heilman, Safran, and Geschwind (1971) of a consecutive series of closed head injuries admitted to the Boston City Hospital, the estimated base rate of aphasia after blunt head trauma is about 2%. Although the exclusion of patients with intracranial operations (other than evacuation of acute subdural hematoma) may have led to an underestimate, a similar study of 1,544 consecutive closed head injury admissions in Bucharest found an almost identical base rate of aphasia (Arseni et al., 1970). The findings of Heilman, Safran, and Geschwind (1971) indicate that frank aphasic disorder occurs only rarely after closed head injury. However, more recent studies (Levin, Grossman, and Kelly, 1976b), employing standardized language tests, have shown that expressive and receptive abilities are frequently impaired after severe closed head trauma. These findings suggest that "subclinical" or "minimal" aphasia is a common sequel of closed head injury. In the early stages of recovery of head-injured patients, confusion and memory disturbances are generally present and may interfere with language processes even in the absence of a classical aphasia typically associated with focal lesions of the dominant hemisphere. Geschwind (1964) characterized this condition as a nonaphasic disorder of speech.

Studies of aphasia after closed head injury have differed considerably with respect to selection of patients, time between injury and assessment, and inclusion of serial examinations to characterize the clinical course. Sarno (1980) has emphasized the difficulty in comparing studies because of these differences. Nevertheless, research on aphasia after closed head injury has disclosed a rather distinctive pattern of speech and language disturbance, which suggests a characteristic course of recovery.

Language during the early stage of recovery

Investigators have only recently plotted the early recovery of communicative skills after prolonged coma in patients with severe closed head injury. In a longitudinal study of 135 patients who were initially unresponsive to commands for at least two weeks while hospitalized on a neurosurgery service, Bricolo, Turazzi, and Feriotti (1980) found that the capacity to obey simple commands was the major milestone in passing through a stage of vegetative state to a relatively normal level of functioning. The ability to obey commands was often delayed after spontaneous eye opening and restoration of a sleep-wake cycle. Occasionally, patients concurrently exhibited vigilance and could obey commands after emergence from coma, but this was atypical. Figure 1-14, from the paper of Bricolo, Turazzi, and Feriotti (1980), depicts the delay in following commands in comparison with spontaneous eye opening, as determined over a six-month period. Of the patients who eventually followed commands, 87% were able to do so within three months after injury and 98.5% by the end of the sixth month.

The appearance of speech following restoration of the capacity to obey commands is also shown in Figure 1-14 of Chapter 1. The period between the second and fourth months postinjury was the peak interval for resumption of speech. Of the patients who eventually spoke during the 12 months of the study, 98.5% did so by six months. At the end of one year, 31% of this series were severely disabled, 8% were persistently vegetative, and 11.5% had succumbed to complications of which bronchopneumonia was the most common.

Najenson, Sazbon, Fiselzon, Becker, and Schecter (1978) also have plotted recovery curves for communicative skills during the first 18 months after severe closed head injury in 15 patients with prolonged coma (undefined). Insofar as these patients were referred to a rehabilitation unit, they were not a consecutive series of severe head injuries admitted to a neurosurgery service as were the patients in the study of Bricolo, Turazzi, and Feriotti. The authors used an innovative scale (Table 7-1) to rate expressive and receptive functions because the patients were unable to cooperate in the standardized tests that are usually employed during the later stages of recovery. Six patients in this study remained in a vegetative state, and nine cases showed partial or full restitution of language.

Table 7-1. Assessment of communication functions after prolonged coma [a]

Auditory comprehension	Oral expression
Awareness of gross environmental sounds	Voicing
Awareness of speech	Saying vowels
Ability to indicate Yes and No	Saying consonants
Understanding own name	Saying own name
Recognition of family names	Saying nouns
Understanding simple verbal orders	Saying verbs
Recognition of names of familiar objects	Saying noun–verb combinations
Recognition of colors	Saying short sentences (automatic)
Recognition of forms	Saying short sentences (non-automatic)
Understanding use of familiar objects	Conversational speech
Visual comprehension	Reading
Awareness of visual stimulation	Reading own name
Understanding gesture direction	Reading family names
Association of identical objects	Reading single words
Association of identical forms	Reading simple sentences
Association of similar objects	Reading newspaper headlines
Categorization	Reading newspaper articles
Speech	Writing
Articulation	Writing own name
Respiration	Writing family names
Voice	Writing words
	Writing simple sentences
	Writing a letter

[a] From Najenson, T. et al. (1978). Recovery of communicative functions after prolonged traumatic coma. *Scand. J. Rehab. Med.* 10:15–21. Reproduced with permission of the authors and publisher.

Najenson and his coworkers observed a consistent sequence of recovery. Comprehension of gestures and oral language first appeared, usually between three weeks and five months after trauma. Oral expression, reading, and writing were slower to recover and motor defects in speech (e.g., articulation, respiratory control, and phonation) were often permanently impaired. Of the nine patients who recovered communication, eight had dysarthric speech. The authors observed that the recovery of communicative ability corresponded to a progressive improvement in locomotion.

The assessment of language during the period of resolving posttraumatic amnesia is complicated by confusion that, in the presence of a mild aphasic disturbance, may give the appearance of a severe language disorder. Inappropriate, fragmented, and tangential speech may occur without impressive anomia or impairment of comprehension. Although it is advisable to concurrently measure orientation while evaluating language during the course of recovery, few have done so. Conversely, expressive language disturbance may give the false impression of confusion on a verbal test of orientation unless the results are verified by using a multiple choice format. In general, the rate of language recovery during this early period is greater than the more gradual improvement over the first year (Kreindler et al., 1975).

The results of early clinical examination for aphasia obtained in consecutive closed head injury admissions at the Boston City Hospital were reported by Heilman, Safran, and Geschwind (1971). Of the total series, the authors found 13 cases of aphasia, including nine patients with anomic aphasia and four patients with Wernicke's aphasia. The authors defined anomic aphasia as a fluent aphasia in which the patient demonstrates verbal paraphasia for all kinds of material, and especially to confrontation. Wernicke's aphasia was defined as a fluent aphasia with paraphasia, impaired comprehension for spoken and written language, and poor repetition. Broca's aphasia was defined as nonfluent aphasia with relatively intact comprehension. The authors' definition of anomic aphasia corresponds to the amnestic aphasia described in other studies (Thomsen, 1975, 1976). No patient had a Broca's aphasia or exhibited total disruption of language. As noted above, the authors excluded patients on whom intracranial surgery had been performed (other than evacuation of subdural hematoma); this selection may have excluded aphasic patients with mass lesions. In contrast to the patients described in other studies of posttraumatic aphasia, the aphasics described by Heilman and his coworkers were older (mean age 57) and nearly one-half were alcoholic.

In a similar study of 26 closed head injury patients without mass lesions who had been in coma for at least 24 hours, Thomsen (1975) found that aphasic symptoms were present during the first two or three weeks after injury in 12 cases. Verbal paraphasia (i.e., substitution of inappropriate words) and anomia were the most common findings. Receptive impairment and dysgraphia were also frequently observed, whereas paragrammatism and other symptoms suggestive of Broca's aphasia were rarely seen. In a related study, Thomsen (1976) found that focal left hemisphere mass lesions were associated with "multisymptomatic" aphasia; anomia, agraphia, and impaired comprehension were common; one-third of the patients with focal left hemisphere lesions had global or receptive aphasia; and anomic aphasia was present in four patients. Consonant with the findings in patients with diffuse closed head injury, symptoms of Broca's aphasia were rare. Among the patients with mass lesion, primary involvement of the left temporal lobe was strongly associated with aphasia.

Morsier (1973) described 23 head-injured patients who had speech or language disturbance or both. Although there is meager information concerning the findings in the total study population from which the aphasic cases were selected, and the interval between injury and assessment is not reported, this study is instructive because it shows a wide range of disturbances. Whereas 11 patients were aphasic, Morsier found diverse language disturbances in 12 additional patients and ten patients had anarthria or dysarthria. Seven cases were dyslexic, six were dysgraphic, four developed posttraumatic stuttering, and three were dyspraxic. He found no relationship between the duration of coma and the persistence of language deficit. This analysis, however, combined the data on patients who had left hemisphere mass lesions with findings obtained in cases of diffuse closed head injury. In contrast to the classical criteria for aphasia used by Heilman, Safran, and Geschwind (1971), Morsier considered a wide spectrum of language and speech disorders.

In a comprehensive study of posttraumatic aphasia, Alajouanine, Castaigne, Lhermitte, Escourolle, and Ribaucourt (1957) attempted to correlate the site of lesion with aphasia both in patients with missile wounds of the brain and in those with blunt head trauma producing focal contusions or posttraumatic thrombosis. It was found that the correspondence between locus of lesion and type of aphasia was consistent with the clinicopathologic correlations established for patients with vascular lesions. Mutism, jargon, alexia, and agraphia were observed in the closed head injury patients, whereas Broca's aphasia was more common in patients with missile wounds of the brain. A more rapid recovery of language was characteristic of the traumatic patients as compared to patients with cerebral vascular disease.

Levin, Grossman, and Kelly (1976b) gave the Multilingual Aphasia Examination (Benton, 1967) to a consecutive series of young adults, with closed head injuries of varying severity who had regained normal orientation. Table 7-2 shows the findings and indicates that defective performance on the Visual Nam-

Table 7-2. The frequency of linguistic deficit assessed by subtests of the Multilingual Aphasia Examination in comparison with the findings of gross aphasia in a series of 50 patients with closed head injury of varying severity°

Findings	n	% of group
Gross Aphasia		
Expressive	1	2
Anomic	1	2
Receptive	0	0
Mixed	6	12
Defective Performance		
Visual Naming	20	40
Sentence Repetition	2	4
Word Association	10	20
Writing–Dictation	5	10
Token Test	16	32
Aural Comprehension	8	16
Reading Comprehension	6	12

°Based on the data from Levin, H.S. et al. (1976b)

ing subtest (e.g., naming line drawings of familiar objects such as a piano) was far more common than the presence of aphasic disorder as diagnosed on the basis of conversational speech or receptive language ability. Circumlocution and paraphasic errors, which were not obvious during a brief conversation, were often disclosed by the testing.

An illustrative case follows.

A 20-year-old, right-handed man was admitted to The University of Texax Medical Branch with a severe closed head injury (Glasgow Coma Scale score 5), but no focal motor deficit. The CT scan suggested generalized brain swelling without a mass lesion. Baseline assessment four months after injury disclosed anomic errors that deteriorated into jargon (e.g., the handle of a fork was called a "forkline" and the calf of the leg was called the "legline"). Circumlocution was evidenced by his response when the examiner pointed to the pedals of a piano—"If you want a different sound, push them down." Word finding was defective on the test of controlled word association.

This patient's findings were representative of the overall results. Table 7-2 indicates that rapid retrieval of words beginning with a specific letter (controlled word association) was frequently impaired in this series. This defect could not be attributed to gross confusion. As suggested by other authors (Groher, 1977; Sarno, 1980), residual memory deficit and persistent difficulty in naming and word retrieval may be expressions of a common underlying deficit resulting from disproportionate injury to the temporal lobes.

Long-term recovery of language

Thomsen (1975) administered a follow-up (mean interval of 31 to 33 months after injury) language examination of her own design to 12 patients who had been aphasic after diffuse closed head injury. Four patients, including two left-handers, showed no signs of recovery of language. In the others, amnestic aphasia, word-finding difficulty, repetition of words or phrases, verbal paraphasia, and perseveration were frequently present. Thomsen noted a residual decline in complex verbal skills such as detailed verbal description and the use of antonyms, synonyms, and metaphors. Impaired reading was found in four cases, but no patient was totally alexic. Although her findings are not incompatible with the view that aphasia secondary to closed head injury generally has a good prognosis (Alajouanine et al., 1957), Thomsen emphasized that residual defects in language analysis and dysarthria were present. Moreover, she pointed out that the manifestations of "subclinical" language problems depend on the recovery of memory and general cognitive function.

In a second study, Thomsen (1976) reexamined the language of 15 patients with focal mass lesions (in which temporal lobe damage predominated) or extensive destruction of the left hemisphere who had been aphasic during the initial hospitalization. When tested at least one year after injury (mean interval 29 months), there was an overall trend of improvement though all patients exhibited residual language deficit. The course of recovery was characterized by improved comprehension of oral and written language and less severe agraphia. In contrast, amnestic aphasia and perseveration persisted in nearly all patients. Global aphasia with gross impairment of all language functions typically evolved into receptive aphasia, whereas patients who initially had a receptive aphasia frequently showed improvement in comprehension. Their findings at the time of followup were compatible with anmestic aphasia.

Thomsen concluded that nearly all patients with focal left hemisphere lesions improved somewhat. She cautioned, however, that "half the patients had severe or moderate aphasia two and one-half years after the trauma and a few had not been able to pass the level of automatic language" (e.g., expletives, stereotyped phrases).

Groher (1977) gave the Porch Index of Communicative Ability to 14 closed head injury patients at one-month intervals beginning shortly after termination of coma (mean of 17 days). Progressive improvement in expressive and receptive skills over a four-month period was the rule. Naming to confrontation recovered in all patients, whereas errors in spelling and syntax and incomplete sentence construction persisted. The degree of recovery suggested by this study appears to be considerably greater than the impression conveyed by other investigators of aphasia after severe closed head injury. It is conceivable that left hemisphere mass lesions were not present in Groher's series, although this is difficult to ascertain because details of the injuries were not described.

Sarno (1980) combined the methods of clinical examination of language and quantitative assessment in a study of a consecutive series of 56 closed head injury patients referred to the Institute of Rehabilitation Medicine in New York. In contrast to some other studies, patients with mild injury were not included. Focal mass lesion or severe depressed skull fracture accounted for about one-half the cases. From clinical observations, Sarno differentiated the series into groups of aphasia (n 18), dysarthria and subclinical language disorder (n 21), and subclinical aphasia (n 17). The diagnosis of aphasia required the presence of unequivocal impairment of expressive or receptive language during conversation, i.e., signs of classical aphasia.

"Subclinical aphasia" denoted defective language processing as reflected by defective scores on the Neurosensory Center Comprehensive Examination for Aphasia (Spreen and Benton, 1966) in patients without signs of aphasia in their conversational speech. The classification of aphasia included fluent (n 7), non-fluent (n 7), anomic (n 2), and global (n 2). The aphasia examination was administered after a median interval of seven months postinjury. Sarno plotted the mean scores of the three groups of patients as percentiles in reference to published test norms for aphasics (Figure 7-1). Normal performance on a subtest would correspond to the 90th percentile or higher on this scale. Although Figure 7-1 shows that language deficit was most severe and pervasive in the aphasic patients, Sarno found an impairment on at least one subtest in every patient. Consonant with the results of the study of Levin, Grossman, and Kelly (1976b), repetition of sentences was relatively preserved in patients with subclinical aphasia, whereas word fluency (controlled word association) was reduced in nonaphasic patients.

Setting aside the issue of whether patients with subclinical language deficit are "truly aphasic," Sarno concluded that "the boundaries which usually help identify and classify patients with linguistic deficits after brain damage do not seem to hold to the same degree for the head trauma patients as they do in the stroke population." The broad categories of language outcome proposed by Sarno (Figure 7-1) should be useful for depicting the results in other series of head injuries.

Recovery from aphasia after an interval of at least six months after closed head injury was investigated by Levin, Grossman, Sarwar, and Meyers (1981) in 21 patients. The results of initial CT and findings from surgery disclosed

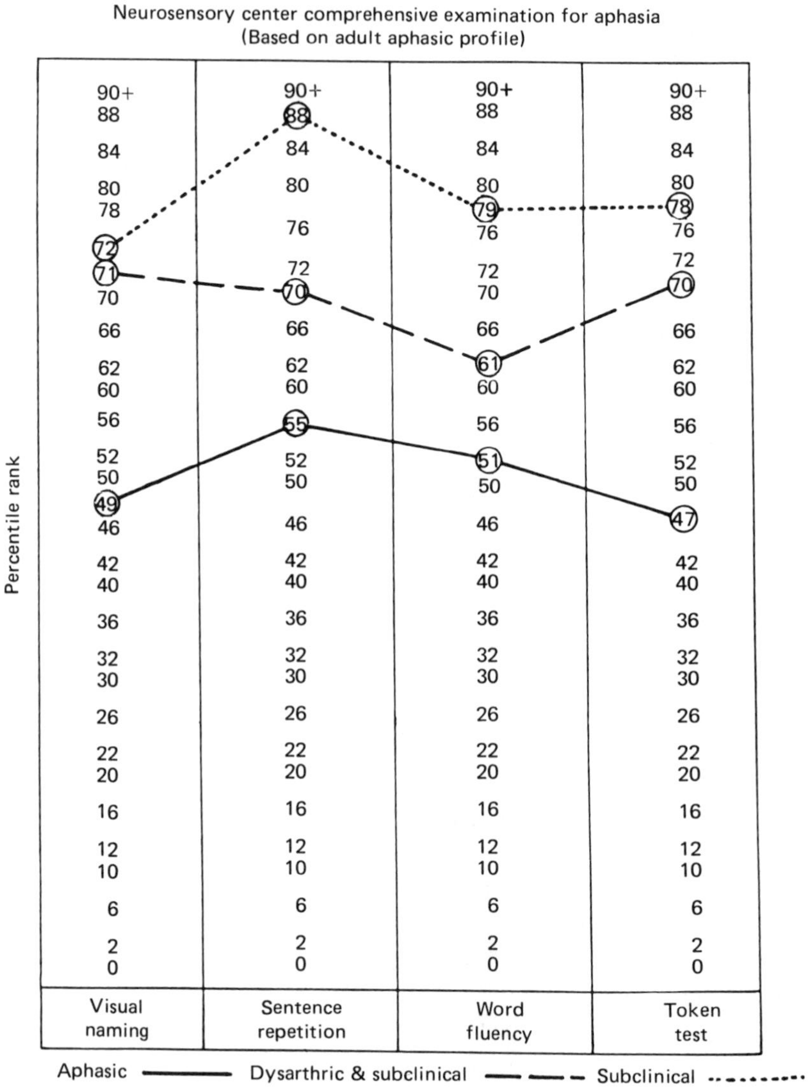

Neurosensory center comprehensive examination for aphasia
(Based on adult aphasic profile)

Fig. 7-1. Mean percentile rank of aphasic and subclinical language disorder groups on subtests of the Neurosensory Center Examination for Aphasia. [From Sarno, M.T. (1980). The nature of verbal impairment after closed head injury. *J. Nerv. Ment. Dis.* 168:685–692. Reproduced with permission of the author and publisher.]

evidence of primary left hemisphere injury in eight cases, focal lesions of the right hemisphere in four cases, bilateral injury in two cases, and diffuse injury in seven cases. The Multilingual Aphasia Examination and portions of the aphasia battery of Spreen and Benton were administered at the time of followup. Nine patients fully recovered from acute aphasia as reflected by uniformly normal scores and intact conversational speech. The 12 patients with residual language deficit (indicated by at least one grossly defective score) were equally divided between those with a persistent impairment of both expressive and receptive abilities and cases of more specific language deficit. Anomia and decreased word finding were the most common isolated defects. Patients who had recovered fully from acute aphasia or who exhibited a specific language disturbance at the time of followup were generally functioning within the average range of intelligence, whereas patients with generalized language impairment evidenced intellectual deficit on both the Verbal and Performance sections of the WAIS.

In contrast to the study of Thomsen (1975) showing that global aphasia after closed head injury evolved into Wernicke's aphasia, in the Galveston series, this transition frequently resulted in a specific anomia. This pattern is illustrated by the serial findings in a 17-year-old student (Figure 7-2A) who had a left temporal mass lesion accompanied by mild to moderate severity of diffuse injury. She initially exhibited impairment of naming, word association, and alexia, whereas residual language deficit was confined to anomia. In contrast, Figure 7-2B depicts persistent, generalized language defects in a 19-year-old patient who sustained a severe closed head injury (coma of 21 days) complicated by bilateral frontoparietal subdural hematomas. He evidenced a concomitant decline in cognitive ability, as reflected by a disparity between followup results on the WAIS and his high school test scores.

In summary, the studies of long-term recovery of language show an overall trend of improvement that may eventuate in restoration of language or specific defects in naming or word finding in about two-thirds of patients who are acutely aphasic. Generalized language deficit, which is associated with global cognitive impairment, persists in patients who sustain severe closed head injury.

Nonaphasic disorders of speech

The neurogenic speech disorders that may occur without aphasia include dysarthria, mutism, echolalia, palilalia, stuttering, and nonaphasic misnaming. When they are present in a nonaphasic patient, there is no evidence of language defects in spontaneous speech, i.e., word-finding disturbance, anomia, agram-

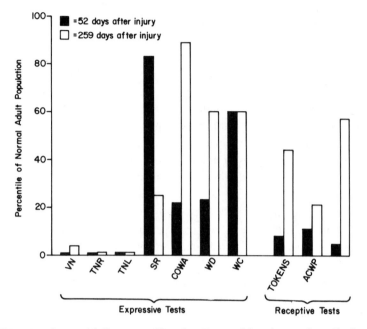

Fig. 7-2A. Baseline and followup profiles of a 17-year-old student with residual anomia that was initially accompanied by a receptive impairment after surgical evacuation of a left temporal intracerebral hematoma. [From Levin, H.S. et al. (1981). Linguistic recovery after closed head injury. *Brain and Language* 12:360–374. Reproduced with permission of the publisher.]

matism, and impaired comprehension (Geschwind, 1964; Weinstein and Keller, 1963). Although this distinction may be obvious in cases of dysarthria, it is difficult in patients who commit errors in naming to confrontation.

Mutism

Total abolition of speech may occur after coma in adults during the transition between spontaneous eye opening and recovery of orientation. As shown in Figure 1-14, the return of speech typically follows comprehension of commands. Prolonged, if not permanent speechlessness is characteristic of patients who are persistently vegetative, who exhibit akinetic mutism (see Chapter 3), or who show findings compatible with the "locked-in syndrome" described by Plum and Posner (1980).

Akinetic mutism (Cairns, 1952; Plum and Posner, 1980) is a form of persisting mutism with little or no vocalization. Behaviorally, this condition is distinguished from the vegetative state by its immobility. The salient features of akinetic mutism include apparent wakefulness with restoration of the sleep-wake cycle and inability to demonstrate cognitive function through interaction with the environment. In general, akinetic mutism has been attributed to lesions that interfere with reticular-cortical or limbic-cortical integration, but that largely spare corticospinal pathways (Plum and Posner, 1980). Large bilateral, basal-mediofrontal lesions of the orbital cortex and adjacent structures have been implicated, as have small lesions interfering with the reticular formation

Fig. 7-2B. The baseline and followup findings in a 19-year-old student show persistent impairment of expressive and receptive language that was associated with cognitive deficit and progressive ventricular enlargement. He sustained a severe diffuse injury (coma of 21 days) complicated by bilateral frontal subdural hematomas. (VN, Visual Naming; TNR, Tactile Naming, Right Hand; TNL, Tactile Naming, Left Hand; SR, Sentence Repetition; COWA, Controlled Word Association; TT, Token Test; ACWP, Auditory Comprehension of Words and Phrases; RC, Reading Comprehension; WD, Writing to Dictation; WC, Writing–Copying). [From Levin, H.S. et al. (1981). Linguistic recovery after closed head injury. *Brain and Language* 12:360–374. Reproduced with permission of the publisher.]

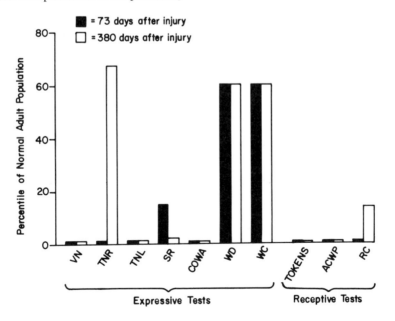

of the diencephalon and adjacent midbrain. When akinetic mutism is a sequel to closed head injury, diffuse cerebral injury is to be suspected.

Locked-in syndrome occurs in quadriplegic patients with bulbar and facial paralysis who have relatively well preserved consciousness and are often able to communicate with residual eye and lid movement (Plum and Posner, 1980). This condition may be distinguished from akinetic mutism and persistent vegetative state on the basis of the preserved capacity for language comprehension and communication with the environment. Traumatic locked-in syndrome can result from direct injury to the ventral pontomedullary junction (Britt, Herrick, and Hamilton, 1977).

Geschwind (1974) distinguishes between nonaphasic and aphasic mutism. The aphasic type, which rarely occurs (cf. Morsier, 1973), is accompanied by linguistic errors in writing. Nonaphasic mutism is associated with acute onset of right hemiplegia; writing is normal and there are no signs of aphasia when speech is restored. Following Bastian (1898), Geschwind refers to this condition as aphemia rather than aphasia. In such cases, mutism may arise from a focal lesion.

In contrast to speech disorder in head-injured adults, an extended period of mutism is common in children with acquired aphasia following head trauma. Hécaen (1976) has described the features of aphasia in children in whom closed head injury was the predominant etiology. Of nine children with left hemisphere mass lesions, six had a period of mutism; of four children with aphasia secondary to a right hemisphere mass lesion, two were mute, and two of the three children with bilateral mass lesions exhibited mutism. The period of mutism varied from five days to three months. Among the children in whom the site of mass lesions could be documented by surgical findings, anterior lesions (frontal or Rolandic) were most common. Four cases with temporal lobe lesions, including a child with concomitant brain stem involvement, were also initially mute. Hécaen observed that the period of mutism was frequently followed by articulatory disturbance, which, however, was usually mild. In other respects, the overall recovery of speech and language was more impressive than the clinical picture seen in adults with aphasia.

In his discussion of the localization of lesions in mute adults, Geschwind (1974) implicated lacunar infarcts of the basal ganglia. Two adolescents with posttraumatic mutism and hemorrhagic contusions of the basal ganglia have been studied in Galveston. The case with the longer period of mutism is summarized below.

A 12-year-old, left-handed girl (with a familial background of some degree of sinistrality) was evaluated 20 minutes after sustaining a closed head injury on 22

June 1979 when she was struck by a car. Examination in the emergency room disclosed a Glasgow Coma Score of 6; she began to obey commands on 30 June, but had a right hemiplegia and uttered no words or sounds. The CT scan disclosed a hemorrhagic contusion of the left putamen and anterior limb of the internal capsule (Figure 1-11). She remained mute until 15 July. Throughout the mute period she was dysgraphic and her spelling, using block letters, was impaired. A repeat CT scan showed changes in density suggesting resolution of the hemorrhagic lesions in the basal ganglia. Detailed assessment of language on 13 August, when she was fully oriented, disclosed an impoverished lexical stock with infrequent initiation of spontaneous speech. The Multilingual Aphasia Examination showed a decrement in verbal associative fluency as well as defective comprehension (Token Test). Spontaneous speech was grossly intact when she was examined a year later. The followup tests disclosed a residual impairment in verbal associative fluency (controlled word association) and impaired comprehension of complex commands (Token Test), although some improvement had been made.

Echolalia and palilalia

Echolalia is the repetition of words spoken by others; palilalia is the automatic repetition of one's own words. Echolalia may follow a period of mutism in cases with diffuse cerebral dysfunction. It may also occur in patients with transcortical motor aphasia who show disturbed conversational speech with preserved capacity for repetition. These disorders also have been observed in patients with large frontal lesions. According to Geschwind (1974), they are uncommon in patients with lesions primarily involving the peri-Sylvian region of the dominant hemisphere.

Stengel (1947) differentiated what he called automatic and mitigated forms of echolalia. Automatic echolalia is parrot-like repetition with no elaboration of the input. Mitigated echolalia is the *questioning* repetition of words spoken by others, often with a change in the personal pronoun. He postulated that mitigated echolalia may facilitate comprehension in patients with receptive language disturbance. Thus, an observed transition from automatic to mitigated echolalia may be a sign of clinical improvement. Stengel also pointed out that the mitigated type may be confined to social conversation and be less evident when the patient is directly questioned by an unfamiliar speaker.

In his series of 50 patients with severe closed head injury, Thomsen (1976) reported echolalia in three cases. Of the two echolalic patients with left hemisphere mass lesions, one initially had a global aphasia and the other had little spontaneous speech. The third patient, who had sustained a severe diffuse closed head injury with residual hydrocephalus, evidenced both echolalia and palilalia. In contrast to the general association of echolalia with impoverished spontaneous speech (cf. Geschwind, 1974), Thomsen commented that the patient with diffuse closed head injury "talked almost constantly without any inhibition."

Echolalia developed after emergence of speech in a young woman admitted to The University of Texas Medical Branch after severe closed head injury. This 18-year-old, right-handed student was brought to the emergency room shortly after an automobile accident on 11 May 1980. Initial examination disclosed a Glasgow Coma Scale of 6, fixed and dilated pupils, and a right hemiparesis. A CT scan on the day of injury was normal. She slowly improved and eventually followed commands on 9 June. She was transferred to the Del Oro Rehabilitation Hospital in Houston on 16 June where she remained confused and disoriented until 26 June. During this period, the patient's spontaneous speech changed from an overall impoverishment to a greater than normal flow in which automatic echolalia was prominent. Observations by Dr. Mary Ellen Hayden and Dr. Ron Levy during the course of rehabilitation showed a transition to mitigated echolalia, which resolved by the middle of July. Repetition was most evident in the presence of persons familiar to the patient. Aphasia examination on 16 July disclosed intact spontaneous speech and almost normal naming. The echolalia had disappeared, but repetition of sentences and verbal associative fluency were still markedly impaired. Comprehension of complex commands on the Token Test was also defective, but the patient could read and understand single words and phrases. Further progress in rehabilitation was complicated by her uninhibited (e.g., sexually explicit) behavior, a finding in agreement with Stengel's interpretation of echolalia as a failure of inhibitory control. At the time of a followup examination ten months postinjury, she exhibited a specific reduction in verbal fluency on the Controlled Word Association Test (Multilingual Aphasia Examination), although her conversational speech was normal.

In summary, echolalia and palilalia are uncommon sequelae of closed head injury. They are apparently confined to cases with severe diffuse injury or large mass lesions in the dominant hemisphere. The absence of any reference to echolalia and palilalia in several studies supports the impression that they rarely occur after closed head injury (Levin et al., 1976; Najenson et al., 1978; Sarno, 1980).

Dysarthria

Sarno (1980) defines dyarthria as a speech disorder arising from pathological alterations of the motor speech system that is evident in defects of the acoustic aspects of the speech stream (i.e., articulation, resonance, stress, and intonation). The severity of dysarthria varies from mild articulatory imprecision to completely unintelligible speech. Dysarthria may be due to a lesion of either the central or peripheral nervous system. Peacher (1945) reviewed the cases of dysarthria recorded by U.S. Army hospitals during World War II. Of the injuries producing dysarthria, which were primarily missile wounds of the brain, 69% involved a lesion of the peripheral nerves. Trauma to the facial nerve was the most common site of lesion, although Peacher did not distinguish between central and peripheral facial nerve injuries.

Investigators of speech disorder after closed head injury have consistently reported dysarthria in patients with focal mass lesion of the left hemisphere (Alajouanine et al., 1957; Morsier, 1973; Thomsen, 1975) and in patients with diffuse cerebral injury (Sarno, 1980; Thomsen, 1976). Dysarthric patients are frequently hemiparetic and sometimes quadraplegic. Serial assessment of language after severe closed head injury has suggested that dysarthria often accompanies aphasia during the early stage of recovery, and it may persist after the restoration of language capacities. This dissociation is illustrated in a patient admitted to The University of Texas Medical Branch, Galveston.

A 33-year-old, right-handed carpenter sustained a severe closed head injury in a motorcycle accident on 17 December 1977. Evaluation in the emergency room shortly after injury disclosed a Glasgow Coma Scale score of 4. A CT scan showed a large left parietotemporal epidural hematoma, which was evacuated on the day of admission; his neurologic condition progressively improved and he followed commands on 20 December. A left facial palsy and right hemiparesis remained. He was moderately aphasic and severely dysarthric, which rendered his speech unintelligible. By the first week in January, the patient's speech improved, although he continued to evidence anomia and impaired comprehension. A CT scan (ten months postinjury) disclosed a large hypodense area at the site of the operated hematoma and a small hypodense area in the genu of the left internal capsule that was interpreted as a small lacunar infarct. He was transferred to a rehabilitation center prior to neuropsychological evaluation, but returned a year later for testing. Speech was fluent, but moderately dysarthric with frequent articulatory defects. Expressive and receptive language skills, however, had uniformly recovered as reflected by normal scores on all subtests of the Multilingual Aphasia Examination.

In contrast to the findings in this patient, Sarno (1980) reported that subclinical language deficit (e.g., decreased word fluency, anomia) was present in all dysarthric patients in her closed head injury series. The findings in the Galveston patients suggest that the correspondence between language skills and motor speech may vary depending upon the interval between injury and assessment.

From these studies, we may conclude that assessment of dysarthria should be included in followup testing of closed head injury patients. The brief tests for articulatory agility and rating speech characteristics in the Boston Diagnostic Assessment Battery (Goodglass and Kaplan, 1972) are useful for this purpose.

Nonaphasic misnaming

Weinstein and Kahn (1955) described patients with brain damage of diverse etiology, including diffuse cerebral disturbance, and lesions of the diencephalon or brain stem, who exhibited misnaming that was qualitatively atypical for aphasia. Errors in naming were associated with objects that were related to the patient's illness (e.g., "spinning wheels" for wheelchair) and personal problems. Nonaphasic misnaming was frequently associated with disorientation, denial of illness, and confabulation. In contrast, Weinstein and Keller (1963) found that anomic errors in patients with left hemisphere lesions (mostly vascular and tumor cases) included phonemic confusion, semantic similarity, and spatial/temporal contiguity. Orientation was often unaffected in these patients. Weinstein and Kahn observed that patients exhibiting nonaphasic misnaming frequently showed no evidence of groping for words, or alteration of speech prosody nor did their naming necessarily improve when correction was offered. Heilman et al. distinguished the anomia in their closed head injury patients from nonaphasic misnaming (Weinstein and Kahn, 1955). In contrast to the narrow range of anomic errors (e.g., related to illness) in cases of nonaphasic misnaming, the anomic head-injured patients described by Heilman et al. exhibited diverse naming defects in spontaneous speech and writing. Six of the anomic aphasics had concomitant defects of higher cortical function including dyslexia, right-left confusion, dysgraphia, and dyscalculia.

Observations of closed head injury patients treated in Galveston who exhibit misnaming suggest that there are individual differences in the type of naming errors and their behavioral correlates. Moreover, the severity of misnaming may differ according to the stage of recovery. Posttraumatic amnesia may accentuate the type of errors reported by Weinstein and Kahn; defective naming in the disoriented patient may not qualify as a classical aphasia.

The anomic disturbance in patients with recent closed head injuries described by Heilman, Safran, and Geschwind (1971) appeared to be similar to that found in patients with focal lesions of the dominant parietal area. Moreover, unequivocal anomic aphasia has been found within three months of closed head injury in Galveston despite precautions against testing language during posttraumatic amnesia. Analysis of anomic errors recorded in followup testing of Galveston patients who had been acutely aphasic has shown a predominance of semantic errors (e.g., "foot" for ankle), circumlocution (e.g., "you push them to make music" for piano pedals), and concrete examples (e.g., "orange" for circle). From the foregoing, it appears that it may be an overgeneralization to presume that all naming errors after closed head injury, even in cases with no focal lesion of the dominant hemisphere, are of the nonaphasic type.

Clinicopathologic correlations

Diffuse injury

Investigators have traditionally employed the duration of coma as an index of diffuse injury severity. Analysis of the relationship between coma duration and resultant aphasic defects has been complicated by the presence of concomitant mass lesions that vary in their localization. Depending on the involvement of the left hemisphere speech area in different series of closed head injury patients, the effects of coma duration may be more or less impressive. The effects of the injury-assessment interval may also depend upon the presence and locus of mass lesion. Patients emerging from a brief period of coma who have an acute aphasia secondary to a dominant hemisphere hematoma may be expected to show rapid recovery of language after resolution or surgical evacuation of the mass lesion. In contrast, patients with a language disturbance associated with severe widespread ischemic necrosis and injury to the white matter (Strich, 1956, 1970) may recover more slowly.

Several investigators have reported no relationship between duration of coma and the severity or persistence of language disturbance (Morsier, 1973; Groher, 1977; Sarno, 1980). The findings on patients with mass lesions, however, are typically merged with those on diffuse closed head injury cases, and there is wide variation in the injury–test interval. Levin, Grossman, and Kelly (1976b) assessed language after resolution of posttraumatic amnesia in young adults, although the interval was longer in patients tested at the time of their clinic visit. Analysis of groups of patients divided according to duration of coma disclosed an overall relationship to residual aphasia. Correlations between coma duration and scores on language subtests, however, were not consistently significant.

From the foregoing it may be predicted that the correlation between coma duration and recovery of language may increase in the long term, whereas the effects of mass lesion are diminished over time. Levin et al. (1981) examined the language of closed head injury patients (tested at least 6 months postinjury) who had been acutely aphasic. The authors found that patients with persistent impairment of both expressive and receptive abilities had had longer durations of coma; the Spearman rank order correlations were impressive, particularly for visual naming ($r = -0.76$) as shown in Figure 7-3. Although there is a suggestion of linearity in the data of Figure 7-3, naming scores in patients with a left hemisphere hematoma tended to be below that of patients with right hemisphere mass lesions. Correlations with duration of coma were also impressive for comprehension of oral language and reading.

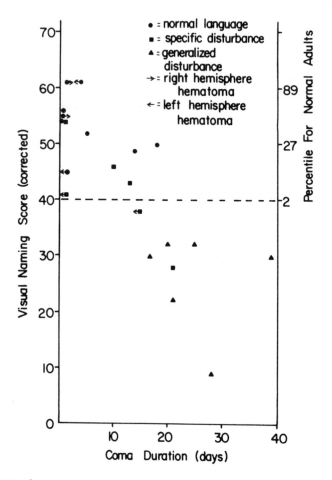

Fig. 7-3. Visual naming scores corrected for age and education plotted against duration of coma for patients with specific linguistic defect, generalized aphasia, and normal language. [From Levin, H.S. et al. (1981). Linguistic recovery after closed head injury. *Brain and Language* 12:360–374. Reproduced with permission of the publisher.]

Severity of generalized injury may also be reflected by acute CT findings of ventricles and cisterns compressed by cerebral swelling (shown in Figure 1-6A in Chapter 1). Of 21 cases with acute aphasia after closed head injury studied by Levin, Grossman, Sarwar, and Meyers (1981), there were three patients who had initial CT evidence of generalized brain swelling with no mass lesion. One of these patients is described below.

A 20-year-old, right-handed student sustained a severe closed head injury on 30 September 1977. The Glasgow Coma Scale at the time of admission on the day of injury was 5; CT findings showed generalized brain swelling. The patient was unable to obey commands until 21 October; he was disoriented and confused until the end of November. Baseline assessment on 4 April 1978 disclosed fluent speech with occasional word finding difficulty. Speech content was impoverished and predominated by stereotyped comments and banalities. Naming to confrontation disclosed paraphasic errors with jargon (e.g., "legline" for calf of leg), semantic approximations (e.g., "zero" for ellipse), and circumlocution (pedals of a piano were described as "if you want a different sound, push them down").

The lack of CT evidence for a dominant hemisphere lesion in patients with brain swelling in no way precludes the possibility that small lesions involving the speech area could be identified by postmortem examination.

Focal mass lesions

In investigations of closed head injury patients with focal mass lesion involving the speech area, the type of aphasia is similar to that evidenced by patients with nontraumatic vascular lesions in corresponding regions (cf. Alajouanine et al., 1957). Left temporal intracerebral hematoma has been confirmed in head-injured patients with fluent, paraphasic speech and impaired comprehension and in a patient with transient alexia with agraphia (Debray-Ritzen et al., 1977; Stone et al., 1978). Dominant temporal lobe injury or more extensive left hemisphere damage accounted for three-fourths of the aphasic closed head injury patients with focal lesions studied by Thomsen (1976).

Heilman, Safran, and Geschwind (1971) observed that external evidence of trauma to the right orbitofrontal region was more common in aphasic closed head injury patients than in nonaphasic patients with head trauma. The authors inferred that contrecoup injury to the opposite hemisphere was responsible. Neuropathologic studies in Glasgow (Adams et al., 1977) have since suggested, however, that contrecoup lesions are less frequent than previously supposed and may not be a major mechanism of brain damage in closed head injuries.

Hemispheric disconnection syndromes

The pathophysiology of closed head injury, which is reviewed in Chapter 1, entails shearing and stretching of axons and resultant injury to the corpus callosum. Although severe closed head injury would be expected to interrupt fiber tracts and produce disconnection syndromes, few investigators have systematically examined this possibility. Goldstein (1942) postulated that transient apraxic disturbances were common during the initial stage of recovery, but were often overlooked.

The earliest description of a hemispheric disconnection after closed head injury was the case reported by Lhermitte, Massary, and Huguenin (1929) of a jockey who developed alexia without agraphia after falling off a horse. He had a right homonymous hemianopsia and a left inferior quadrantanopsia. The patient could not read words, but could read single letters. A second study of hemispheric disconnection after closed head injury was published 40 years later by Schott, Michel, and Michel (1969), who described a patient with tactile anomia, ideomotor apraxia, and agraphia confined to the left hand. There was no anatomic confirmation of injury to the corpus callosum.

The first report of cerebral hemispheric disconnection after closed head injury with neuropathologic verification described a 50-year-old, right-handed alcoholic who had sustained a right basilar skull fracture and developed a right subdural hygroma after a fall (Rubens et al., 1977). Examination shortly after a later left frontal infarction (14 years after injury) disclosed borderline cognitive functioning, but no aphasia. In contrast to preferred and superior performance with his left hand on a nonverbal motor test (e.g., pegboard), he was unable to produce a single correct left-handed movement (e.g., gesture, imagined use of object) in response to verbal command nor did he benefit from example. However, he correctly demonstrated the use of real objects with his left hand. Agraphia was confined to his left hand, although copying designs was less affected. Autopsy findings five months after the behavioral study showed marked thinning of the corpus callosum with demyelination and loss of axons. Injury to the corpus callosum extended from the posterior one-third of the genu to the midsplenium. White matter injury was also evident in both cingulate gyri, the fornices, and the mammillary bodies. Rubens et al. concluded that the disconnection syndrome may have been potentiated by the later frontal infarct and the focal lesions to the right hemisphere at the time of injury, but that the initial injury to the corpus callosum was primarily responsible.

In a study of long-term recovery from acute aphasia after closed head injury, Levin, Grossman, Sarwar, and Meyers (1981) tested interhemispheric transfer of information by comparing the naming of objects placed in the left or the right hands. They found a disproportionately severe impairment in naming objects placed in the left hand, a finding they viewed as evidence for callosal dysfunction. Two patients with residual expressive and receptive deficits also exhibited ideomotor apraxia in that they could do no better than approximate familiar gestures on oral command. Followup CT showed ventricular enlargement in both patients, although there were no clinical signs of obstructive hydrocephalus or delayed cognitive deterioration. Consistent with neuropathologic studies of closed head injuries (Strich, 1956, 1970), ideomotor apraxia may have resulted from initial shearing and stretching of axons and degenerative changes in the white matter affecting intrahemispheric connections.

Summary

Aphasia is clinically evident in a relatively small proportion of closed head injury patients. It is more likely to occur in cases with mass lesions involving the dominant hemisphere and in patients with severe diffuse injury. Subclinical language disturbance, as reflected in poor verbal memory and impoverished verbal associative fluency, is fairly common after closed head injury but may require quantitative tests to be documented. Anomia, decreased word finding, and impaired comprehension of complex commands may be present in patients without obvious aphasia. Of the nonaphasic disorders of speech, dysarthria is the most frequent and may occur with aphasia or in isolation.

The prognosis for recovery from aphasia after closed head injuries in young adults is generally better than in cerebral vascular disease, although it varies with the severity of overall cerebral injury. Persistent language deficit is closely associated with general cognitive impairment. Symptoms of hemispheric disconnection after severe injury may be present more often than has been previously thought; its diagnosis requires assessment of writing, ideomotor praxis, and tactile naming.

8. Perceptual and motor skills

Neuropsychological studies of soldiers with penetrating missile wounds of the brain have documented the presence of visuoperceptive deficit, impaired performance on such visuomotor tasks as tracing a maze with a manually guided stylus, and somatosensory defects on tests of punctate pressure sensitivity and two-point discrimination (Corkin, 1979; Newcombe, 1969; Semmes et al., 1960). Systematic study using similar procedures to assess the effects of closed head injury has been relatively meager in most areas of sensorimotor performance and visual perception. Effort has hitherto been directed toward measuring reaction time in closed head-injured patients (Miller, 1970; Van Zomeren and Deelman, 1978). Visual perception has also been considered in a few studies. In general, however, the effects of severe closed head injury on sensory and motor abilities have been largely unexplored by neuropsychological techniques.

Reaction time

Retardation in speed of response is commonly found in patients with brain damage arising from vascular disease or neoplasm (cf. Blackburn and Benton, 1955). The degree of retardation in reaction time is directly related to the complexity of the task, which is typically determined by the number of equiprobable visual or auditory signals that are discriminative for different response keys or buttons (Dee and Van Allen, 1973). The finding that retardation of response speed increases as a function of task complexity has been interpreted as evidence for slower decision-making in patients with cerebral disease (Dee and Van Allen, 1973).

Miller (1970) studied simple and complex visual reaction times in five young adults who were tested between three and 12 months after closed head injuries that produced a period of posttraumatic amnesia of at least one week. In comparison with a control group, the severity of psychomotor retardation in the head-injured patients increased with the number of equiprobable stimulus lights (one, two, four, or eight), which signaled the response to corresponding buttons. In view of Miller's findings, it may be postulated that serial measurement of reaction time in which there is a decision posed by different response locations would more closely reflect long-term recovery from severe closed head injury than would simple reaction time, i.e. an invariant response to the same key corresponding to a light in a fixed location.

Strong support for the employment of choice reaction time as an index of severity of closed head injury was provided in a longitudinal study of 57 severely injured young men who were hospitalized in Groningen (Van Zomeren and Deelman, 1978). The patients were divided into mild, moderate, and severe injury groups according to the duration of coma (less than 16 minutes, less than seven days, over seven days), which was defined as a total Glasgow Scale score of 8 or less. The initial test was given after clearing of posttraumatic amnesia, which persisted for less than one week in the mildly injured patients and for more than four weeks in the severely injured patients. Serial reaction time studies performed over a period of two years after injury disclosed evidence of a progressive reduction, which was significantly greater in patients who had prolonged periods of coma (Figure 8-1 A,B). It can be seen in Figure 8-1B, however, that reaction time in patients two years after severe injury was still slower than the reaction time of 90% of the subjects in a control group. Figure 8-1B also shows that the improvement in response speed over two years was most impressive on a four-choice reaction time task, whereas a relatively flat recovery curve (Figure 8-1A) was found for simple reaction time (one light, one button). Choice reaction time measured at five months after closed head injury correlated significantly with the Glasgow Coma Scale score obtained on the sixth day of hospitalization, duration of coma, and clinical outcome rated on the Glasgow Outcome Scale, 12 months postinjury. The authors interpreted these findings as compatible with the view that impaired information-processing capacity is a persistent sequel of severe closed head injury.

Retardation in response speed on a complex reaction time task was also demonstrated by Gronwall and Sampson (1974) in patients tested within 24 hours of mild closed head injury (no coma or mass lesion). Reaction time had

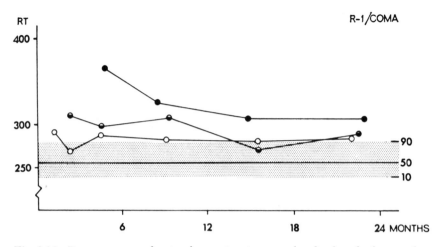

Fig. 8-1A. Recovery curves for simple reaction time, as related to length of coma after injury. Shaded area below indicates the normal range of a non-injured reference group. On the abscissa, number of months after injury is plotted. ●, group with coma longer than one week; ○, group with coma between one hour and seven days; ○, group with less than 60 minutes. [From Van Zomeren, A.H., and Deelman, B.G. (1978). Long-term recovery of visual reaction time after closed head injury. *J. Neurol. Neurosurg. Psychiat.* 41:452–457. Reproduced with permission of the authors and publisher.]

Fig. 8-1B. Recovery curves for choice reaction time as related to length of coma after injury. Symbols as in Figure 8-1A. [From Van Zomeren, A.H., and Deelman, B.G. (1978). Long-term recovery of visual reaction time after closed head injury. *J. Neurol. Neurosurg. Psychiat.* 41:452–457. Reproduced with permission of the authors and publisher.]

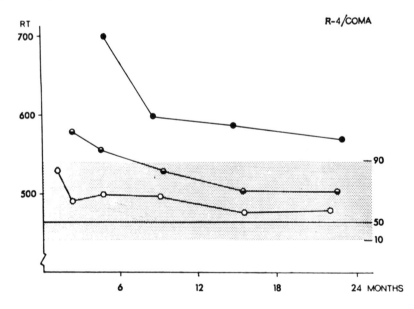

improved markedly when the patients were retested a month later. The finding of a similar, albeit transient, impairment of information processing in their series is consonant with the view that the effects of "concussion" differ quantitatively rather than qualitatively from those of severe diffuse closed head injury.

The design of apparatus and testing procedures employed in these reaction time studies hold the range of movement constant under the simple and choice reaction time conditions. Thus, it is plausible to attribute the greater sensitivity of the latter task to a reduction in the rate of information processing in head-injured patients.

The authors of these studies restricted testing to patients without focal motor weakness, a precaution that strengthens an interpretation emphasizing slowed information processing. Further study is necessary to elucidate the mechanisms of injury that primarily contribute to slowed response speed.

Halstead-Reitan tests

An investigation of recovery from closed head injury in children using an adaptation of the Halstead-Reitan battery, by Klonoff and his associates, is summarized in Chapter 10 (Klonoff, Low, and Clark, 1977; Klonoff and Paris, 1974). One hundred adults who sustained a head injury within 24 months of examination were given the Halstead-Reitan battery modified by Kløve and Cleeland (1972). Although it is not entirely clear from their report, this study was apparently restricted to cases of closed head injury. Figure 8-2 shows that patients with abnormal findings on neurological examination within a month of injury exhibited a more impaired neuropsychological profile than patients with no neurologic deficit. As seen in Figure 8-2, the WAIS Performance Scale IQ and arithmetic ability (Wide Range Achievement Test) were closely related to neurologic findings, as was the Tactual Performance Test, a task that involves placement of geometric shapes into a formboard without the aid of vision. In addition to recording the time required to correctly insert the blocks using each hand on separate trials, the test also includes a measure of retention of the specific shapes and their respective locations on the board. Duration of coma, i.e., the period from injury to the point in time when the patient first obeyed verbal commands, was negatively correlated with adequacy of performance when this test was given more than six months after injury. Performance on the Halstead Categories Test, a nonverbal problem-solving test that stresses abstracting ability, was also related to coma duration. Detailed analysis suggested that three weeks was a critical duration of coma, in that decrements in performance were most impressive when coma persisted beyond this point.

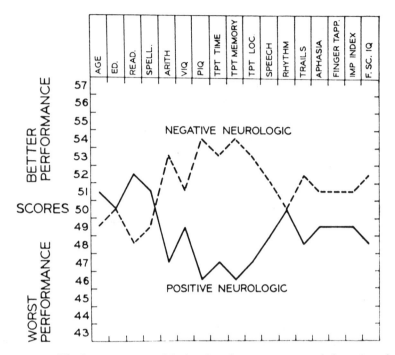

Fig. 8-2. Profile of T-scores on modified Halstead-Reitan neuropsychological test battery contrasted for patients with negative and positive neurologic findings. In patients tested four months or longer after injury, the neurologic examination was performed within one week of testing and at least 48 hours after the patient had regained consciousness. [From Kløve, H., and Cleeland, C.S. (1972). The relationship of neuropsychological impairment to other indices of severity of head injury. *Scand. J. Rehab. Med.* 4:55–60. Reproduced with permission of the authors and publisher.]

There was a trend for patients who had an intracranial hematoma removed surgically to exhibit more severe neuropsychological deficit than other closed head injury patients. Although test scores were generally depressed in patients with a hematoma, significant differences were confined to the Performance Scale IQ and the Trailmaking Test, a timed procedure in which the patient draws a line to connect a scattered array of circles in numeric sequence (Trail A) or alternating between numeric and alphabetic sequences (Trail B). The Impairment Index, a composite measure of the proportion of tests comprising the battery with defective scores, was related to the presence of asymmetric weakness or reflex changes on neurologic examination within a month of injury. Support for the prognostic significance of the Halstead-Reitan battery administered during the early phase of recovery is provided by the results of Dikmen and Reitan (1976), who assessed long-term outcome at 18 months. An initially severe neuropsychological deficit was predictive of persistent disability. In contrast to the earlier study by Kløve and Cleeland (1972), there was no analysis of neurologic indices of initial injury severity.

In summary, the series of tests comprising the Halstead-Reitan battery have been shown to reflect the severity of closed head injury. The WAIS Performance Scale, Categories Test, Tactual Performance Test, and Trailmaking Test are among the most sensitive variables comprising the battery. In view of the frequent finding of residual memory deficit as described in Chapter 5, it would be advisable to supplement the Halstead-Reitan battery with tests of memory.

Visual perception

Vulnerability of the visual pathways to craniocerebral trauma was demonstrated by Crompton (1970) in necropsy studies of 84 consecutive patients dying shortly after acute closed head injuries. This series had a bimodal (15–20, 55–60 years) age distribution and was evenly divided between vehicular and domestic accidents. Crompton reported that ischemic necrosis and shearing lesions of the intracranial portion of the optic nerve predominated with less frequent involvement of the optic foramen and optic chiasm. Hemorrhagic lesions of the visual pathways were unrelated to the presence of intracranial mass lesion, whereas optic nerve injury was associated with diffuse brain damage. Crompton did not report on retrochiasmal involvement. Chiasmal visual loss in patients surviving closed head injuries with wide variation in duration of coma has been recently reported (Savino, Glaser, and Schatz, 1980).

Visuoperceptive ability was studied by Ruesch (1944a) in "unselected" patients who had recently sustained a closed head injury and in patients with "prolonged posttraumatic syndrome" who had been injured six months or more prior to being studied. Ruesch found that the onset of negative after-images was delayed in the acutely injured patients, but not in chronic cases. Dark adaptation time was relatively unaffected.

Discrimination and retention of faces in brain-damaged patients has engaged the interest of neuropsychologists (cf. Benton, 1980), particularly following published reports of patients with prosopagnosia, an uncommon disability involving a specific inability to recognize the faces of familiar persons. Necropsy findings of prosopagnosic patients have consistently demonstrated bilateral cerebral disease, including a lesion in the territory of the right inferior occipitotemporal region (Benton, 1979a; Meadows, 1974). On the other hand, studies employing the CT scan have described some patients with lesions apparently confined to the right hemisphere (cf. Whitely and Warrington, 1977). The etiology in most cases is vascular occlusion. Visual field defects, particularly involving the upper left quadrant, have been present in nearly all reported cases of prosopagnosia.

Transient inability to recognize close relatives is frequently mentioned by families visiting patients during the transitional stages of recovery from closed head injury. Although such anecdotal reports may reflect the patient's generalized confusion, it is conceivable that diffuse brain swelling and hemispheric disconnection arising from shearing and stretching of axons produce impaired facial recognition.

Prosopagnosia was present for several months after a severe closed head injury (coma of 21 days) in a patient described by Levin and Peters (1976). Although CT was unavailable at the time of this study, skull x-rays, brain scan, and carotid arteriography were performed at a community hospital shortly after injury and were interpreted as normal. Visuospatial impairment, memory deficit, and hypersexuality were associated with his failure to recognize family members and close associates. Visual fields were full and his prosopagnosia had cleared when he underwent a neuropsychological examination one year after injury; verbal ability had recovered satisfactorily despite residual visuospatial deficit (Verbal IQ = 101, Performance IQ = 79).

From the analysis of cases of prosopagnosia, investigators have developed tests to assess discrimination, matching, and memory of photographs of unfamiliar faces (cf. Benton and Van Allen, 1968; Warrington and James, 1967). These studies have shown that impaired ability to discriminate unfamiliar faces frequently occurs in patients with brain disease, particularly in cases with posterior right hemisphere lesions. Hamsher, Levin and Benton (1979) found that impaired recognition of unfamiliar faces in patients with unilateral left hemisphere disease was confined to aphasic patients with receptive language deficit. Among patients with preserved language comprehension, defective facial recognition was specifically related to right hemisphere involvement. More than one-half of the patients with post-Rolandic right hemisphere lesions were affected. Visual field defect was related to impaired recognition of unfamiliar faces, although full fields in affected cases were more common than in prosopagnosic patients (Meadows, 1974).

On the basis of studies of facial recognition in patients with focal brain lesions, similar findings might be anticipated in patients with closed head injuries complicated by right hemisphere hematoma. Levin, Grossman, and Kelly (1977a) assessed the recognition of unfamiliar faces in 46 such patients, including six cases with intracranial hematoma. The 27-item short form of the facial recognition test (Levin, Hamsher, and Benton, 1975) was given after orientation had reached a normal level or at least had substantially improved. The test consists of three sections including (1) matching identical front-view photographs of a face, (2) matching a front-view with profiles from different angles, and (3) matching front-view photographs under varying light conditions. Defective facial recognition performance (i.e., a score below that of 97% of control patients) was found in more than one-quarter of the closed head injury patients who had been comatose for periods over a few minutes. Only two patients (17% of the mildly injured cases) with coma limited to a few minutes exhibited impaired recognition of unfamiliar faces. Of the patients with an intracranial mass lesion, facial recognition deficit was restricted to two patients with an intracerebral hematoma situated in the right hemisphere, although four additional patients with right hemisphere hematoma achieved normal scores. Of interest was the finding of residual impairment of facial recognition in a patient with a right posterior parietal intracerebral hematoma who was unconscious for only several minutes and fully responsive at the time of hospital admission. This case illustrates a specific neuropsychological deficit probably attributable to a circumscribed lesion complicating an otherwise mild closed head injury.

Although visuoperceptive deficit is not widely regarded as a salient feature of the neuropsychological profile after closed head injury, this study suggests that subtle deficits of this type may occur.

Tachistoscopic perception

Tachistoscopic presentation allows precise control of duration to assess the capacity for identification of brief stimuli. This procedure provides an opportunity to determine the minumum duration required for processing discrete information with no demands on response speed. Underlying the application of the tachistoscope is the assumption that the perceptual capacity of head-injured patients may be adequate for stimuli presented under normal conditions, but not for stimuli that are briefly presented. This possibility was confirmed by Ruesch (1944a), who compared tachistoscopic perception in recently head-injured patients with that of patients who had sustained a closed head injury at least six months previously. Three-digit numbers were presented in central vision at increasing exposure durations varying from 20 msec to 1 sec. The author found that the minimum exposure duration necessary for identification of the numbers was increased by 33% in previously injured patients and by 142% in more recently injured (but unconfused) patients as compared to a control group. Of interest was the finding that the threshold duration (lower duration indicative of more efficient processing) could be correlated with the Wechsler-Bellevue IQ ($r = -0.41$) in recently injured patients, whereas age was a major determinant ($r = 0.56$) of performance in the "chronic" closed head injury group. In contrast to more recent neuropsychological studies, the average age of both closed head injury groups exceeded 35 years. From these data Ruesch inferred that the delayed processing in recently injured patients was "an expression of intellectual impairment." There was no relationship between the threshold duration and such neurologic signs as pathologic reflexes, cranial nerve palsy, and the presence of bloody spinal fluid (examination of cerebrospinal fluid was commonly performed at the time of the study).

The lack of correlation between tachistoscopic threshold duration and specific neurologic findings led Ruesch to conclude that "delayed apperception may be an expression of minor or diffuse brain damage," although he cautioned that the elevated threshold in closed head injury patients may have been influenced by disturbances of attention and fatigability. The results convincingly demonstrated a delay in processing discrete stimuli under controlled conditions and suggest the usefulness of tachistoscopy in outcome research.

Tachistoscopic perception was recently investigated by Hannay, Levin, and Kay (1981) in 51 patients who were examined after a closed head injury of varying severity (median interval of 14 months). Cases with a visual field defect were excluded from this study. The test stimuli were three letters arranged vertically and presented to the left or right visual field after termination of a 2 sec central fixation dot. This method permitted selective stimulation of either visual field prior to a saccadic eye movement. It was postulated that severe generalized closed head injuries would delay processing of briefly presented stimuli as a consequence of injury to the cerebral white matter and that involvement of the corpus callosum would particularly disrupt recognition of letters flashed to the left visual field. The latter prediction was based on the assumption that recognition of verbal material presented to the left visual field requires interhemispheric transfer of information for analysis by structures in the left hemisphere specialized for reading.

Letter trigrams were initially presented in central fixation to estimate the minimum duration necessary for correct identification. Patients with mild closed head injury, i.e., those who were alert on admission with no neurologic deficit, did not differ overall from more severely injured patients in their threshold duration (the median was about 20 msec), although five patients with severe injury failed to identify letters in central vision until the duration was at least 50 msec. Recognition of letter trigrams presented to either visual field at threshold duration (but increased by a constant) was impaired in patients with severe as compared to mild closed head injury. Significant differences obtained when severity was defined according to the duration of coma as measured by the period in which the patient was unresponsive to simple commands. Contrary to prediction, the degree of deficit was generally comparable in the left and right visual fields. The results confirmed a delay in processing discrete chunks of information without imposing a time limit on the patient's response, as is the case with Paced Auditory Serial Addition. It is conceivable that this perceptual delay reflects the extent of degradation in transmission of information within the cerebral white matter. It is also possible that slowed tachistoscopic perception in these patients may represent a subtle form of hemispheric disconnection.

Summary

Efforts directed toward characterizing the neuropsychological outcome of closed head injury have been concentrated on intelligence and memory with relatively few investigations of perceptual and motor skills. Studies published to date have confirmed that retardation of response speed persists after severe injury and that performance on complex reaction time and perceptuomotor tasks is frequently impaired. The discrimination of faces and the identification of tachistoscopically presented stimuli are also sensitive to the residual effects of closed head injury. Focal hematoma involving the right hemisphere contributes to visuoperceptive deficit. Somatosensory and auditory functioning following closed head injury have yet to be systematically investigated.

9. Psychiatric consequences

Behavior disturbances after head injury were recognized as early as the 16th century, when Fabry reported that head injuries may cause "insanity." Although early descriptions did not include clinicopathologic correlations, the authors reported a wide spectrum of behavioral sequelae in their patients. At the turn of the century, Adolf Meyer (1904) described a series of head-injured patients who developed "posttraumatic insanity," which he characterized as a syndrome of neuropsychological and psychiatric deficits. Many current classification schemes provide for the categories of posttraumatic psychosis, neurotic reactions, including the posttraumatic or "post-concussional" syndrome, and posttraumatic personality disorder. The third edition of the Diagnostic and Statistical Manual for Mental Disorder (DSM-III) of the American Psychiatric Association specifies the "Organic Personality Syndrome" in which head trauma is among the most common etiologic factors. According to DSM-III, there is a marked change in behavior or personality involving at least one of the following: (1) emotional lability (e.g., temper outbursts, sudden crying); (2) decreased impulse control (e.g., poor social judgement, sexual indiscretions); (3) marked apathy and indifference; and (4) suspiciousness or paranoid ideation.

Studies of recovery from closed head injury, however, suggest a wider range of posttraumatic psychiatric disorder. The classification employed in the following discussion attempts to take account of this variety. Some diagnostic terms are used for descriptive purposes without the implication that they are necessarily equivalent to the use of these terms for psychiatric disorders with other etiologies.

Psychiatric manifestations of closed head injury may be broadly classified according to their time of onset with respect to the injury and the patient's overall level of consciousness. Acute psychiatric disturbance occurs during the transition from coma to reorientation and may persist for days or weeks thereafter. Residual chronic psychiatric effects may continue after termination of posttraumatic amnesia. They may progressively diminish until the patient is considered "back to normal," or they may produce a permanent alteration of behavior, i.e., an enduring change in personality from the preinjury condition. Stern (1978) has elaborated three phases of psychiatric disturbance after head injury; the first phase begins with recovery of consciousness, the second is the subacute phase, which begins when the acute symptoms remit, and the third corresponds to relatively permanent changes in personality, which represent residual changes. The following section is organized according to the predominant symptoms, though phases of recovery are distinguished in a scheme similar to that described by Stern.

Acute posttraumatic psychosis

Behavioral effects during the initial hospitalization for head injury are observed both in patients who are confused and stuporous, but not comatose at any time, and in patients during various stages of emergence from coma to orientation. Early behavioral manifestations cover a wide range of severity. Depending on the symptoms present, subtypes of posttraumatic psychosis have been described as "schizophrenic-like," Korsakoff's psychosis, depressive psychosis, manic-depressive psychosis, paranoid psychosis, and reactive psychosis (Hillbom, 1951). In 1922, Hadley reviewed consecutive head injury admissions of military personnel to the Walter Reed Hospital in which both closed head injuries and penetrating missile wounds were represented. Although Hadley and later Hall (1925) accepted the primacy of neurologic injury in producing a transient psychosis, they concluded that preinjury personality traits were largely responsible for the failure of a psychotic state to resolve. Consequently, Hadley argued for "delimitation of material" in selecting patients for future studies. Of 1,821 brain-injured soldiers examined by Hillbom at varying intervals after penetrating missile wounds of the brain or closed head injuries, 81 (4.5%) were psychotic. Selection criteria (e.g., severity and type of injury, preinjury characteristics) for defining a study sample have varied among previous authors and thus variation across studies concerning the risk of posttraumatic psychosis is to be expected.

Schizophrenic-like psychosis

The designation "schizophrenic-like" reflects the florid disorganization of thought evidenced by incoherent speech, tangential associations, and inappropriate thought content. Hallucinations may occur in any modality; data bearing on the relative frequency of auditory, visual, and tactile hallucinations after head injury are unavailable. Lishman (1973) inferred from his review of the head injury literature that when major psychosis follows head injury, "constitutional predisposition is undoubtedly the major factor." But not all investigators agree with his inference. Hillbom (1951) found that posttraumatic psychosis with schizophrenic-like symptoms was associated with evidence of temporal lobe damage to which he attributed the occurrence of hallucinations and seizures. Hillbom asserted that only a very small proportion of these patients showed evidence of preinjury schizoid personality. Viewed from the perspective of recording admissions to a state psychiatric hospital, Shapiro (1939) estimated that about one-half of the posttraumatic admissions were considered to have "latent" preinjury emotional disorder or a vulnerability. The other patients with posttraumatic schizophrenia were reported by Shapiro to have no signs of preexisting psychiatric problems; brain injury, as reflected by neurologic deficit, seizures, and prolonged coma were more strongly implicated in this latter group. Posttraumatic schizophrenic symptoms following closed head injury in patients transferred to psychiatric institutions have been confirmed by other authors (Alliez and Somani, 1967; Guyotat et al., 1968). Guyotat, Dumas, and Marie-Cardine (1968) and Shapiro (1939) reported that head injury was temporally contiguous with the onset of schizophrenic symptoms in 1.6% and 1% of psychiatric admissions, respectively.

Acute confusional state

Moore and Ruesch (1944) described prolonged disturbance of consciousness after closed head injury that frequently occurred as patients emerged from periods of coma of varying duration. They called attention to exceptional cases who evidenced severe confusion for periods exceeding three weeks, despite relatively brief durations of coma; acute agitation or traumatic delirium was noted to occur immediately in some patients. According to recently established criteria based upon coma scales (cf. Teasdale and Jennett, 1974), many of these patients had transient periods of coma or never lost consciousness. Disorientation for time and place was the most persistent feature in the series studied by Moore and Ruesch. It was often accompanied by fluctuating vital signs (pulse, temperature, and respiration). Increased psychomotor activity, incoherent talkativeness, agitation, aimless movements, and inappropriate actions were frequently noted. Hallucinations were comparatively rare. Of the neurologic correlates, the presence of an EEG abnormality was most closely associated with persistent confusion, a finding reported in 93% of their patients. Interpretation of the findings reported by Moore and Ruesch in terms of causal relationships is complicated by their lack of selection criteria for patients in the study. More than one-half of their cases had a preinjury history of psychiatric disorder and/ or alcoholism. Chronic alcoholism was associated with persistence of confusion after head injury.

Confabulation, i.e., a fictitious narration of past events or distorted version of an actual occurrence, is frequently present during an acute confusional state (Weinstein and Lyerly, 1968). Confabulations frequently involve other people (both real and nonexistent), the circumstances of injury or reasons for hospitalization (which Weinstein and Lyerly described as confabulations about personal violence in brain-injured soldiers), or the circumstances of work and occupation. Reduplicative delusions (reproductive paramnesia) for place, person, and time were also prominent in the patients studied by Benson, Gardner, and Meadows (1976) and by Weinstein and Lyerly. This amnestic-confusional condition has been characterized as Korsakoff's psychosis by several authors (Alliez and Sormani, 1967; Guyotat, Dumas, and Marie-Cardine, 1968; Schilder, 1934; Weinstein and Lyerly, 1968). A detailed discussion of amnesic deficit during the subacute phase of recovery is included in Chapter 4. It will suffice to point out here that most patients abandon their distorted interpretations of the injury and surroundings as their orientation returns to a normal level.

Levin and Grossman (1978) confirmed the observations of Moore and Ruesch concerning the confusional state by studying patients after closed head injury in whom there was no history of previous neuropsychiatric disorder including chronic alcohol abuse. Agitation in these patients was manifested by thrashing of extremities, truncal rocking, dislodging intravenous tubes and catheters, yelling, combativeness, and attempts to get out of bed. It has been frequently necessary to physically restrain these patients to prevent further injury. Acute agitation was frequently a prelude to disinhibitory behavior; as the level of confusion partially diminished, overreaction to minimal provocation, uncontrollable laughter without apparent precipitant, and sexually explicit behavior ensued. Agitated and disinhibitory behavior after closed head injury occurred in patients who were heterogeneous with respect to preinjury personality and demographic characteristics. Levin and Grossman (1978) found, however, that the presence of acute agitation was associated with greater residual psychiatric disturbance.

An acute confusional state after closed head injury was reported by Groslambert, Perret, and Boucharlat (1965) in a patient with a right temporal contusion.
The authors suggested that this hemispheric locus of injury was particularly
likely to produce marked confusion. Their contention has received support from
Mesulam et al. (1976), who described acute, nontraumatic confusional states in
three patients with infarctions in the distribution of the right middle cerebral
artery. The authors postulated that corticocortical connections converging on
the inferior frontal, supramarginal, and angular gyri of the right hemisphere
may subserve complex integrative processes involved in selective attention.
Interruption of cortical connections emanating from limbic structures was
implicated by Mesulam et al. in such "psychosis-like behavior" as agitation and
inappropriate actions.

Affective psychosis

In his review of the psychiatric sequelae of closed head injury, Lishman (1973)
asserted that affective psychosis after head injury is much more common than
posttraumatic schizophrenia. He also contended that "the idea of precipitation
in the predisposed person remains unchallenged, and there is little to date to
suggest an additional organic etiology" (page 314). An inherent difficulty in the
psychiatric classification of disorders after head injury is the frequent finding of
an admixture of affective symptoms, thinking disturbance, and hallucinations
(Levin and Grossman, 1978). The incidence of reactive depression after head
injury is less difficult to determine, but it has not been studied systematically.
    During the subacute phase of recovery, affective disturbance can take the
form of euphoria accompanied by a lack of insight regarding the injury and its
resultant neurologic deficits. An unwarranted buoyant mood is usually empty
and unassociated with delusions of grandeur (Shapiro, 1939). Conversation may
convey a sense of excitement, though accelerated speech is usually not present.
Depressive symptoms may be precipitated by misinterpretation or reduplication of the circumstances (e.g., the patient may believe he is incarcerated). In
patients with less severe cognitive impairment, depression may be an appropriate reaction to neurologic injury, multiple trauma, and feelings of helplessness
engendered by awakening confused in a neurologic intensive care unit (Schnaper and Cowley, 1976).
    Levin and Grossman (1978) have reported both hypomanic and depressive
behavior after closed head injury. Against Lishman's postulation concerning the
paramount importance of preinjury personality, they found that the severity of
injury was directly related to the degree of residual affective disorder. Symp-

toms of elation and depression were relatively mild, if present at all, in a comparison group of patients who were spared neurologic deficit and who were awake on admission to the hospital. Studies of neurochemical alterations following closed head injury suggest that disruption of brain catecholaminergic (Van Woerkom et al., 1977; Boismare et al., 1977) and cholinergic metabolism (Grossman et al., 1975) by the injury may trigger the onset of marked affective symptoms.

Prolonged elated and disinhibitory behavior after severe diffuse closed head injury was described by Levin and Peters (1976) in a college student seen ten months after injury (1973) in which he was rendered comatose for three weeks in a community hospital. Neurologic examination a year after injury showed him to be alert, euphoric, cooperative, and well-oriented. Neurologic findings were normal except for a reduced light reaction in the left pupil, anosmia, and minimal clumsiness in hopping. An angiogram performed at the time of injury was normal, as were the serial EEG, brain scan, and skull x-rays at the time of followup; CT was unavailable at the time. The patient complained of inability to assimilate new knowledge adequately. For several months following the injury he was prosopagnosic, i.e., he was unable to recognize his children or his friends. The patient's wife had become alarmed by his diminished social judgement, euphoria, irritability, and hypersexuality. Detailed study of his preinjury history provided no evidence of antecedent neuropsychiatric disorder.

Following the subacute state of injury, modulation of affective expression generally improves, although the residual picture may be one of apathy and indifference. Several authors (Gronwall, 1976b; Levin and Grossman, 1978; Schilder, 1934) have noted that severely injured patients frequently develop affective blunting characterized by a veneer of pleasant, but bland demeanor and a cordiality that obscures a lack of insight regarding their marked deficits. Schilder (1934) linked affective blunting with a residual Korsakoff's psychosis and he commented that "it is astonishing how little the patients are concerned about their head injuries" (pg. 165). Levin and Grossman (1978) observed that this constriction of affective expression is associated with social withdrawal, engagement in such solitary activities as listening to music, and cognitive impairment.

Characteristics of patients who develop posttraumatic psychosis

Narrative notes and ratings on the Brief Psychiatric Rating Scale (BPRS) (Overall and Gorham, 1962) were completed on adults and adolescents who were

Table 9-1. Psychotic behavior during the early stage of recovery from closed head injury

Age	Sex	Initial Glasgow Scale° V	E	M	Coma°° (days)	Initial CT†	Redupl	Manifestations observed during Confab/ delusions	Halluc
20	F	4	4	6	0	WNL		Paranoid fear	Visual
21	M	4	4	6	0	WNL		Having baby	
19	M	2	4	6	0	WNL		Delusions of grandeur; paranoid	
25	M	4	4	6	0	Right sylvian SAH; vertex EH			
27	F	1	1	5	<1	Diffuse swelling		Having baby	Visual; audit
24	M	T	1	5	2	Right insula IH	Geogr	In prison for crime	Audit
18	M	3	1	5	4	Bifront IH	Geogr; context	In army	
24	F	1	1	5	4	Diffuse swelling	Geogr; persons	Having baby, paranoid	Visual
19	M	1	1	4	20	Bifront SH	Geogr	Extraordinary confab of injury; paranoid	
21	M	1	1	2	36	Right temp EH		Circumstances of injury	

Abbreviations: CT, computed tomography; Redupl, reduplication; Confab, confabulation; SAH, subarachnoid hemorrhage; EH, epidural hematoma; IH, intracerebral hematoma; bifront, bifrontal; temp, temporal; geogr, geography; R, restraints required; Disinhib, disinhibition; Exhib, exhibitionistic behavior.
°Glasgow Scale scores obtained on admission to hospital. Abbreviations: T, tracheostomy; V, verbal; E, eye opening; M, motor; explanation of scale is given in Chapter 1.

admitted to the Neurosurgery Service of The University of Texas Medical Branch, Galveston, during the period 1974–1978. These patients were studied prospectively and a number of them were selected for study from a total sample of 800 admissions during this period because of their bizarre behavior. The data for these patients appear in order of coma duration in Table 9-1. Historical information obtained from a relative showed no previous neuropsychiatric disorder, chronic alcoholism, or drug abuse in all but one patient. Patient 7 (Table

initial hospitalization				Initial	Brief Psychiatric Rating Scale‡			Follow-up		
Agitation	Disinhib	TD	HS	WR	AD	TD	HS	WR	AD	Psychiatric sequelae
Extreme hypoact		+	+	++	+	0	0	++	0	Transient lethargy
Screaming; out of bed	R	++	0	++	++	0	0	+	+	Transient uncontrolled laughter
Thrashing; pacing	R	++	++	+	0	0	0	+	+	Psychiatric hospitalization
Motor restlessness	R; exhib	0	0	+	+	0	0	+	+	None
Motor restlessness	R; exhib	++	++	++	+	+	0	0	+	Hypomanic, over 6 mos; decreased insight
Thrashing; screaming	R	++	++	++	Unavailable					None
Motor restlessness	R	++		++	+	0	+	+	0	Disinhibited behavior
Screaming; restlessness	R; exhib	++	+	++	+	0	0	0	+	None
		++	+	+	+	++	0	++	++	Borderline personality
Screaming; empty excitement	R	++	++	++	++	+	+	++	+	Psychiatric hospitalization; poor insight

**Coma duration refers to period during which patient could not respond to commands.
†Initial CT performed within 7 days of injury.
††Median Injury: injury BPRS interval, 19 days; 206 days for injury-follow-up BPRS; TD, thinking disturbance; HS, hostile suspiciousness; WR, withdrawal retardation; AD, anxiety depression; 0, not present; +, mild; ++, moderate to severe.

9-1), who had a history of childhood hyperactivity and truancy with no previous evidence of psychosis and documented average preinjury intelligence, was included because of the significance of his serial CT scans, which showed bifrontal intracerebral hematomas (Sweet et al., 1978). The hematomas gradually resolved without surgical intervention.

Acute psychotic manifestations were primarily characterized (90% of series) by confabulatory and delusional themes, which were frequently fragmented, in contrast to the systematized delusions found in psychiatric patients with para-noid schizophrenia. Persistent fabrication of the circumstances surrounding the injury and hospitalization was often present; paranoid ideation (e.g., of bodily harm) was also common. Hallucinations were clearly present in nearly one-half the group. Most patients were markedly agitated or combative, in which case physical restraints (denoted by "R" in the table) were necessary to prevent fur-ther injury. Reduplicative paramnesia was essentially limited to the belief of being in a different place (e.g., Hawaii). Sexually explicit behavior (denoted by "exhib" in Table 9-1) was also observed.

The profile of behavioral ratings on the BPRS corresponded to the pattern generally found in a large series of patients with severe closed head injury (Levin and Grossman, 1978), although the severity of disturbance was greater in this group. The BPRS ratings after the patient initially regained orientation (median injury-rating interval 19 days) indicated that marked thinking distur-bance, emotional withdrawal, and motor retardation were the most prominent features. Hostility, suspiciousness, anxiety, and depression were less conspicuous. The followup examination (median injury-rating interval 206 days) disclosed an impressive degree of behavioral recovery. Although no patient was considered to be psychotic at the time of followup, several patients had attained only a marginal adjustment, i.e., manifested a posttraumatic borderline personality disorder as described later in this chapter.

The neurologic correlates of posttraumatic bizarre behavior are summarized in Table 9-1. A wide range of coma duration was found. The CT results were abnormal in 70% of the patients studied. Diffuse cerebral swelling and mass effect associated with hematoma were the salient CT findings.

Neurotic sequelae

Neurotic symptoms are the most common psychiatric effects of head injury (Lishman, 1973; Miller, 1961). Neurotic disorder after head injury is generally found in patients recovering from mild injuries that produce only momentary or no loss of consciousness and that may not require hospitalization. Insofar as follow-up neurologic examination of these patients tends to be less intensive than in severe injuries, transient neurotic manifestations are less likely to be recorded. Although there is no consensus regarding the classification of neurotic disorders after head injury, several authors have drawn distinctions among postconcussional or posttraumatic syndrome, accident neurosis, and reactive depression (Lishman, 1973; Miller, 1961).

Miller distinguished postconcussional syndrome from accident neurosis primarily on the grounds that the latter is a nonspecific effect of physical trauma in which injury to the head is only incidental. Similarly, reactive depression may occur in isolation or as a complication of postconcussional syndrome after mild head injury.

Postconcussional syndrome

The postconcussional syndrome refers to a constellation of somatic and psychologic symptoms including headache, dizziness, fatigue, diminished concentration, memory deficit, irritability, anxiety, insomnia, hypochondriacal concern, hypersensitivity to noise, and photophobia. As the term "postconcussional" suggests, these symptoms are most frequently reported in patients with brief periods of coma or otherwise disturbed consciousness. In a recent study of consecutive minor head injuries, Rutherford et al. (1977) found that one-half of the patients evidenced at least one postconcussional symptom six weeks after injury. As discussed in Chapter 1, the concept of concussion as a fully reversible injury with no structural alteration of the brain has been challenged on the basis of histologic observations of the brains of concussed patients who subsequently died of non-neurologic injury (Oppenheimer, 1968). This evidence favors the view of concussion as falling along a continuum of diffuse injury severity.

Among the most informative studies of postconcussional syndrome are those published by Brenner and his colleagues (1944) and Friedman, Brenner, and Denny-Brown (1945). These papers are noteworthy because they were based on a series of 200 consecutive civilian head injuries who were selected within an age range between 15 and 55 years; patients who were chronic alcoholics were excluded. In contrast to these studies, other authors (cf. Miller, 1966) have described postconcussional syndrome in patients who were referred because of persistent symptoms or litigation. The Brenner group focused on the symptoms of dizziness, vertigo, and headache, and reported that one-half of the series complained of brief episodes of dizziness at some time after injury, although persistence of these symptoms after discharge from the hospital occurred in only one-third of the cases. Of the patients with residual dizziness, 76% also complained of headache and two-thirds exhibited symptoms of anxiety or depression. The association between headaches and dizziness has since been substantiated in patients with mild closed head injury (Cartlidge, 1978). In the Brenner study, dizziness persisting beyond two months after injury was associated with a symptom aggregate, i.e., anxiety, decreased concentration, irritability, fatigability, and headache. The incidence of this constellation of symptoms was greater in patients 40 to 55 years old than in those patients who were below 30 years of age. The finding of increased risk of postconcussional symptoms in older patients has also been corroborated (Rutherford et al., 1977). Indeed, Lishman (1973) has commented upon the rare occurrence of these symptoms in children.

Vertigo was found in only 11 patients in the total series. After finding no relation between vertigo and injury of the labyrinth, Brenner and his colleagues conjectured that vertiginous patients may have sustained brain stem injury. In contrast, Cartlidge (1978) reported positional nystagamus in 30% of patients who complained of dizziness at the time of discharge; electronystagmographic (ENG) recordings suggested that dizziness in most cases was of labyrinthine origin. Onset of dizziness after discharge from the hospital was rarely associated with nystagamus or an abnormal ENG.

Brenner and his colleagues (1944) described postconcussional headache in the same series of patients hospitalized in Boston in whom they had studied dizziness. The headaches, which occurred in more than two-thirds of the patients at some time after injury, varied with respect to localization and severity. Only one-third of the series reported headaches beyond two months postinjury and persistent headache was related to pretraumatic neuroticism, litigation, and occupational problems. Unlike dizziness, headaches bore no relation to posttraumatic amnesia, but were related to the presence of scalp laceration at the time of injury and, by implication, reflected a phobic reaction. Persistent headaches were also far more common in patients who were injured in an industrial setting. Concomitant with onset of headaches were fatigue, postural changes, and emotional upset. Recently, Rutherford et al. (1977) reported that headaches were present six weeks after injury in one-quarter of a series of consecutively admitted patients with minor head injuries. In contrast to the early studies in Boston, the authors found a relationship between headaches and reports of decreased concentration and memory, but no other evidence of a cluster of symptoms.

The setting in which a mild head injury occurs evidently contributes to the risk of postconcussional syndrome. Miller (1961) contended that the symptoms are infrequent after injuries occurring in sporting events, whereas they commonly occur following industrial accidents in which litigation is involved. There is, of course, the possibility that athletes may be motivated to minimize postconcussional symptoms so that they can resume their activities. Contrary to Miller's emphasis on litigation as a predominant etiologic factor, Merskey and Woodforde (1972) reported that postconcussional symptoms persisted (median duration four years) after mild closed head injury (coma less than one hour) in a series of 27 patients who either were not seeking financial compensation or had already been awarded a settlement. This group was comprised of patients who were requesting psychiatric treatment, most frequently because of depression and anxiety. Merskey and Woodforde rejected Miller's view of financial gain as a primary motive for persistent postconcussional symptoms. It should be noted, however, that this group was comprised of patients referred for psychiatric treatment and was not a consecutive series of head injuries.

The influence of injury severity on postconcussional symptoms has been disputed. Miller contended that there is an inverse relationship between severity of head injury and the development of postconcussional sequelae. Although Friedman, Brenner, and Denny-Brown (1945) found that dizziness was more common in patients in whom posttraumatic amnesia exceeded 12 hours, headaches in the same series were unrelated to duration of amnesia (Brenner et al., 1944). No relationship between posttraumatic amnesia duration and postconcussional residua was found by Rutherford, Merrett, and McDonald (1977) in patients with mild closed head injury, although the authors acknowledged the inherent ambiguities in measuring posttraumatic amnesia, particularly retrospectively. Although there is no consensus on the question, the most widely held opinion regarding the role of injury severity is that postconcussional symptoms persisting more than two or three months after a mild injury most likely reflect an exacerbation of a previous neurotic condition (Guttmann, 1946; Lishman, 1973).

Evidence suggesting that postconcussional symptoms may arise from cerebral dysfunction derives from studies on acute neurologic findings, efficiency of information processing during the first three months after injury, and measurement of cerebral blood flow. Postconcussional symptoms at six weeks after minor head injury were found by Rutherford, Merrett, and McDonald (1977) to be more common in patients who had previously complained of headaches and diplopia within 24 hours after injury. As described in detail in Chapter 6, Gronwall and Wrightson (1974) found that improvement in serial addition performance paralleled the reduction in postconcussional symptoms in patients studied within several days of mild closed head injury. The recovery curve for paced serial addition provided a useful guide in counseling patients about returning to work. That neuropsychological functioning corresponded so closely to postconcussional symptoms during the early stage of recovery suggests that the latter did not reflect a neurotic predisposition. Further support for the importance of subtle cerebral dysfunction was provided by Taylor and Bell (1966). They found delayed cerebral blood flow in patients with postconcussional symptoms who were studied four to eight weeks after closed head injury that produced no coma and who were not attempting to obtain financial compensation. Although the authors conceded that the slow cerebral circulation time in their patients may have been merely coincidental with the reported symptoms, serial findings confirmed that reduction of the symptoms paralleled the recovery of cerebral blood flow. Increased cerebral vasomotor resistance was postulated as the causal factor in the postconcussional symptoms.

Divergent conclusions regarding the validity and etiology of postconcussional symptoms undoubtedly reflect variation in patient selection, the context (e.g., medicolegal, psychiatric, neurosurgical) in which the patients are studied, and the methods (e.g., interview, neuropsychological, cerebral blood flow) employed by the investigators. Integration of the findings of published studies suggests that postconcussional symptoms that begin shortly after the injury and continue for a period of up to two months may result from subtle neurologic dysfunction as reflected by a transient reduction in cerebral blood flow and information-processing capacity. Prolonged postconcussional symptoms, particularly when they appear only after discharge from the hospital, are more likely to occur in patients with a previous neurotic condition or personality disorder that is intensified by the trauma or by extrinsic factors.

Quantitative assessment of behavioral disturbance

Most studies of behavioral disturbance after head injury have described series of patients in nosological terms and have tabulated various symptoms to characterize the psychiatric effects. Quantitative assessment of behavioral sequelae, however, offers the opportunity to study the effects of neurologic indices of injury severity on dimensions of behavioral functioning that can be analyzed as continuous variables (e.g., severity of disturbance) as contrasted with dichotomous variables (e.g., "present vs. absent"). Perhaps the first detailed report of personality test findings during recovery from closed head injury was that of Benton and Howell (1941). The Rorschach test in combination with other measures disclosed evidence of residual personality alteration and cognitive disturbance in a patient whose course of recovery was serially evaluated.

Of the quantitative personality tests currently employed by psychologists, the Minnesota Multiphasic Personality Inventory (MMPI) is the most widely used, particularly in the United States. The findings on serial examination (initial hospitalization, 12 months, 18 months) by the MMPI in a series of 27 consecutively admitted closed head injury patients were reported by Dikmen and Reitan (1977). They found that the patients with residual neuropsychological deficit were older and evidenced greater somatic concern (Hypochondriasis Scale), depression, and a lower level of energy (Mania Scale) than patients who performed normally on neuropsychological tests. Their conclusion was that previous investigators had underestimated the extent of cognitive deficit (and, by inference, the severity of brain damage) in patients with posttraumatic emotional sequelae. The strategy of Dikmen and Reitan in examining the convergence between neuropsychological impairment and emotional disturbance was innovative. Assessment of such a small series of patients heterogeneous with respect to injury severity and demographic characteristics, however, imposes constraints on the causal relationships that may be imputed in their study. Application of the MMPI is necessarily limited by the requirement of at least a sixth-grade reading level. Thus, patients with a limited educational background may have to be excluded from study as well as severely injured patients with posttraumatic reading disabilities (Levin, Grossman, and Kelly, 1976b). Moreover, sole reliance on the MMPI precludes assessment of personality during the subacute phase of recovery, when behavioral disturbance is most florid.

Levin and Grossman (1978) employed the Brief Psychiatric Rating Scale (BPRS) of Overall and Gorham (1962) to obtain a profile of behavioral disturbance after closed head injury of varying severity. The BPRS consists of 18 scales (Figure 9-1), each of which is rated by the examiner on a scale ranging from one (absence of symptom) to seven (most severe manifestation of symptom). Satisfactory interrater reliability has been established for the scales (Overall and Klett, 1972). The ratings were based on a semistructured interview, unobtrusive behavioral observations, and the patient's behavior during neuropsychological testing and were made only after the phase of acute confusion and disorientation had subsided. Selection criteria included no antecedent history of previous neuropsychiatric disorder and an age limit of 50 years. The injuries were classified as Grade I (n 25) in which the patient was conscious on admission and throughout the period of hospitalization with no evidence of neurologic deficit; Grade II (n 24) in which there was a period of coma for not more than 24 hours with or without neurologic deficit; Grade III (n 21) in which coma duration exceeded 24 hours with or without neurologic deficit. On the average, the BPRS ratings were obtained four weeks after injury in Grade I patients, nearly two months after injury in Grade II patients, and six months after injury in Grade III patients.

Profiles of BPRS scores are depicted in Figure 9-1 according to grade of injury; the grand mean (extreme right side) represents the average score on the 18 scales for each grade of injury. Differentiation of the grades of closed head injury severity by the BPRS was evaluated by analysis of covariance with the injury test interval used as a covariate. It was found that scales measuring emo-

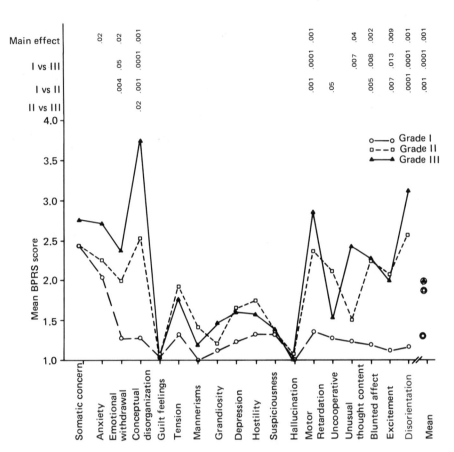

Fig. 9-1. Mean score by each grade of injury on individual scales of Brief Psychiatric Rating Scale (BPRS), with grand mean and results of analysis of covariance. Scale scores were adjusted for effects of variation in the injury-rating interval. Order of scales corresponds to that of the published BPRS. Key: ○—○, grade I; □--□, grade II; ▲—▲, grade III. [From Levin, H.S., and Grossman, R.G. (1978). Behavioral sequelae of closed head injury. *Arch. Neurol.* 35:720–727. Reproduced with permission of the publisher.]

tional withdrawal (e.g., lack of spontaneous interaction, isolation), conceptual disorganization (e.g., disconnected thought processes), motor retardation (e.g., slowed movements and speech), unusual thought content, blunt affect, excitement, and disorientation most efficiently discriminated the patients with respect to grade of injury. Analysis of previously derived clusters of scales (Overall and Klett, 1972) confirmed the initial findings. The factors of Thinking Disturbance and Withdrawal–Retardation both clearly differentiated the grades of injury severity, whereas Anxiety–Depression and particularly Hostile–Suspiciousness were less informative in this regard.

Neurologic indices of acute injury severity were considered in relation to the BPRS findings. The presence of an EEG abnormality, which was predominantly focal or diffuse slow wave activity, was positively related to subsequent Thinking Disturbance and Withdrawal–Retardation. Abnormal CT findings were also related to the behavioral effects as compared to cases with normal CT scans. Limiting the analysis to CT performed within 30 days of injury, it was found that diffuse cerebral swelling as reflected by "slit-like" ventricles was associated with greater residual behavioral deficit. A trend suggesting more severe Thinking Disturbance in patients who developed ventriculomegaly approached statistical significance in the small number of cases affected.

Long-term behavioral disturbance was investigated by using the BPRS at least six months after closed head injury in a series of 27 young adults in whom the initial Glasgow Coma score was 8 or less, i.e., compatible with severe injury (Levin et al. 1979). Chronic socioeconomic dependence (i.e., moderate or severe disability on the Glasgow Outcome Scale) was found in patients who exhibited prolonged Thinking Disturbance and Withdrawal–Retardation. Ratings of Thinking Disturbance were inferred from tangential, fragmented speech not attributable to aphasia and deficient cognitive filtering of irrelevent material. These patients often failed to appreciate the severity of their cognitive deficit and would either focus on relatively minor residual symptoms or deny any sequelae. Slowing of gross movement and speech contributed to the ratings of Withdrawal–Retardation. Mild anxiety and depression on the followup BPRS were also pervasive, but less closely related to general outcome. A review of interview data at the time of followup indicated that complaints of residual cognitive deficit predominated (59% of series). Depressed mood, marital/family problems, and increased anxiety were also common. Followup BPRS ratings in patients who had psychotic episodes triggered by closed head injury are shown in Table 9-1. As in the larger series of patients, the behavioral residua of acute posttraumatic psychosis were cognitive disorganization, withdrawal, and slowed movement.

Summary

The psychiatric effects of head injury encompass a wide range of severity and chronicity. Converging sources of evidence support the view that the postconcussional symptoms and psychosis that emerge during the subacute phase of injury and later subside are the result of varying degrees of brain injury. In the case of postconcussional symptoms, the cerebral dysfunction appears to be at least partially reversible, whereas residual behavioral disturbance is common after psychosis triggered by severe head injury. The potential contribution of alteration of brain neurotransmitters to these clinical pictures is discussed in Chapter 1. The preinjury personality and extrinsic factors, such as litigation, undoubtedly may prolong and intensify symptoms, particularly after minor head injury.

10. Neuropsychological consequences of closed head injury in children

Experimental studies of animals in the 1950s and 1960s produced considerable evidence to suggest that brain damage sustained in infancy did not produce as severe behavioral impairment as did comparable damage in adult animals. For example, Kennard (1938) reported that unilateral ablation of the cortical motor areas in infant primates did not lead to the serious contralateral motor impairment seen in older animals, but only to some loss in fine motor skills. Similarly, ablation of the cortical somatosensory areas in the newborn cat did not produce the tactile deficits observed after the same insult in mature cats (Benjamin and Thompson, 1959). Although it had been demonstrated that mature cats deprived of auditory cortex were unable to discriminate between sounds of different duration or timbre, analogous lesions in infant cats did not result in significant impairment of discrimination (Diamond and Neff, 1957; Scharlock Neff, and Strominger, 1965; Scharlock, Tucker, and Strominger, 1963). Bilateral excision of the striate area, which impairs visual discrimination learning in adult cats, was reported to have no effect on subsequent visual performance in cats operated shortly after birth (Tucker, Kling, and Scharlock, 1968). Nor did bilateral ablation of the prefrontal areas in newborn monkeys produce the "frontal lobe syndrome" characteristic of the behavior of mature animals subjected to the same operation (Akert, Orth, Harlow, and Schlitz, 1960).

Clinical studies of infants and young children were in accord with these experimental findings on animals. There was the century-old observation that congenital or early acquired damage of the left hemisphere does not lead to the aphasic disorders that follow the same damage in adults (Cotard, 1868). Instead, bilateral damage, probably involving brain stem pathways as well as the cerebral hemispheres, seemed to be required to produce specific failure in the development of speech (Benton, 1964; Landau, Goldstein, and Kleffner, 1960). Similarly, acquired aphasia from a brain lesion in a child who had already developed speech was found to be less severe and less permanent than in adult patients (Alajouanine and Lhermitte, 1965; Guttman, 1942). The remarkably mild effects of cerebral hemispherectomy performed on hemiplegic children to relieve epileptic seizures and behavioral disorders provided additional evidence that the behavioral consequences of brain damage were less severe in children than in adults. Both sets of findings support the generalization that the consequences of brain injury are less severe in children, presumably reflecting the greater plasticity in the organization of their central nervous system.

However, more recent investigation of the effects of experimental lesions in young animals and clinical studies of recovery from head injury in children have called into question any simple generalization about "neural plasticity" in the young brain. As will become evident, sparing of function after brain injury depends upon the degree of commitment of the relevant brain structures at the time of injury. The clinical literature suggesting greater capacity of children to recover from focal lesions is clearest for aphasia, but less convincing in other areas. Moreover, there is no impressive evidence indicating that immaturity confers any advantage in withstanding the effects of diffuse cerebral insult. Quite to the contrary, several studies have shown that residual neuropsychological deficits may be more severe after head injury in young children than in adolescents. Direct comparison of outcomes after closed head injury in children and adults is complicated by apparent differences in the pathophysiologic mechanisms of brain injury. Our review draws attention to the need for outcome research that integrates acute neurologic indices including a coma scale, CT findings, and the results of serial administration of neuropsychological tests. Formulation of the characteristic behavioral changes and social sequelae of closed head injury in children must remain tentative until the completion of longitudinal studies that incorporate systematic assessment of behavior and interviews with the family.

Plasticity of the young brain

Experimental and clinical studies have demonstrated distinctive mechanisms of injury and patterns of recovery in young organisms. Early studies by Kennard (1938) showed that ablation of the motor cortex in infant monkeys resulted in relative sparing of motor functions, whereas in contrast corresponding lesions in mature animals produced severe acute impairment. Kennard observed that, as the operated infants matured, they exhibited motor incoordination. Sparing of function after ablations has also been demonstrated in the infant visual and somatosensory systems (Eidelberg and Stein, 1974; Finger, 1978). Nevertheless, limitations in plasticity of function have become increasingly evident. Goldman (1973) has demonstrated that orbitofrontal lesions produce comparable deficits in both young and mature animals on a delayed alternation task, whereas there was apparent sparing after dorsolateral frontal ablation during infancy. Late deficit produced by the early dorsolateral lesions was also found by Goldman, suggesting a variable rate of development for different regions of frontal cortex.

Clinical evidence for plasticity of the young brain has been obtained in studies showing no aphasia when infantile hemiplegia occurs prior to the attainment of language and only transient or mild aphasia when hemispherectomy was performed on young children with hemiplegia who had acquired language prior to surgery (Basser, 1962; Teuber, 1978; Wilson, 1970). Smith and Sugar (1975) have described the development of superior verbal skills in a patient who underwent left hemispherectomy at age 5 because of intractable seizures.

Teuber (1978) qualified the generality of plasticity in finding that undisturbed development of language following perinatal and postnatal left hemisphere damage apparently was achieved with some sacrifice of functions primarily subserved by the right hemisphere. In contrast to these results, he found that early right hemisphere lesions resulted in later visuospatial deficits with no evidence of compensation by greater participation of the left hemisphere. He inferred that an early commitment to language by the left hemisphere, coupled with a subsequent commitment of the right hemisphere to visuospatial functions, might account for the sparing of language and for the vulnerability of nonverbal processes. Aphasia sustained by children after age 10 is more permanent and is consistent with the hypothesis of a gradient of functional commitment of the left hemisphere to language, which increases in slope as the child approaches puberty. Recent evidence suggests that the commitment of the left hemisphere to language may begin as early as the second year of life (Woods and Carey, 1979).

The concept of plasticity has also been weakened as a result of studies of diffuse insult to the young brain due to encephalitis, meningitis, and Reye's syndrome (Davidson, O'Tuama, Willoughby, Swisher, and Benjamins, 1978). Residual cognitive deficit secondary to infection has consistently been more severe when the onset of illness was during early infancy as compared to later in childhood. Similar vulnerability of the immature brain has been suggested with respect to the effects of seizure disorder and malnutrition (Lewis, 1976; Winick, 1976). In summary, although the immature brain may exhibit greater resilience to the effects of focal brain lesions, depending upon the locus of injury and the age of the animal, it may be more susceptible to the effects of diffuse damage than the adult brain.

Epidemiology of closed head injury in children

Accurate incidence and prevalence statistics for closed head injury in children are unavailable because of the lack of a centralized system for case ascertainment. Hospital-based studies in England and Wales have established that accidents account for 16% of all hospital admissions of children under 15 years of age and that more than one-third of all pediatric accident cases and 41% of pediatric mortalities involve head injury (Craft, 1972; Field, 1976; Jamison and Kaye, 1974). In contrast to the predominance of vehicular accidents in producing about one-half of blunt head injuries in adults, road traffic accidents account for one-third of cases of pediatric closed head injury. Falls are responsible for about one-half of the head injuries in children. In comparison with the high incidence of severe closed head injury in young adults who are occupants in vehicles involved in high-speed accidents, pedestrian–car accidents occurring at relatively slow speed are more common in children. It is conceivable that young adults in vehicular accidents are exposed to greater force and thus sustain more severe brain damage due to the acceleration and rotation to which the brain is subjected. Similar to the findings of studies of closed head injury in adults, the epidemiology of pediatric closed head injury indicates a male predominance with a ratio that varies from 2:1 to 3:1 (Craft, 1972; Field, 1976; Hendrick et al., 1964). However, these studies do indicate that the disproportionately high representation of males in closed head injury admissions is somewhat less for children under the age of five years.

In studies of outcome of closed head injury in children, a lower mortality than in adults has consistently been reported (Bruce, Schut, Bruno, Wood, and Sutton, 1978; Craft, 1972; Hendrick et al., 1964). This reflects both studies of consecutive pediatric admissions (Hendrick et al., 1964) and studies in which patients have been selected on the basis of a Glasgow Coma Scale score indicating severe injury. In contrast to a mortality of 30 to 50% in adults with Glasgow Scale scores below 8 (Becker et al., 1977; Jennett et al., 1977), Bruce et al. (1978) report a corresponding figure of only 9% (6% when adjusted for cases of brain death at the time of admission). These statistics agree closely with those based on consecutive head injury admissions to the Hospital for Sick Children in Toronto (Hendrick et al., 1964). Although greater capacity for survival in children after closed head injury is implied, Hendrick, Harwood-Nash, and Hudson (1964) noted that variation in the cause of injury (e.g., more frequent high speed motor vehicle accidents in young adults) may be a contributing factor.

Mechanisms of closed head injury in children

The apparently greater capacity of young children to survive severe closed head injury as compared to adults is not fully understood. A number of anatomic and physiologic features of head injury in children may be contributory (Bruce et al., 1978; Hendrick et al., 1964). For example, the greater flexibility of bones in young children may enhance the capacity of the skull to absorb traumatic forces, thereby lessening focal brain injury (Craft, 1975; Gurdjian, 1958).

Gurdjian postulated that the relatively shallow cerebral convolutions of the young brain would result in greater deformation of the brain on impact, potentiate shearing effects, and contribute to brain stem injury, and accordingly, oculovestibular disturbance and pupillary deficit would occur more frequently in childhood closed head injury. This hypothesis has been supported by the evidence. Bruce, Schut, Bruno, Wood, and Sutton (1978) analyzed in detail the clinical findings of 53 pediatric closed head injury cases who fulfilled the criteria for severe injury according to the Glasgow Scale, i.e., inability to obey commands, utter comprehensible speech, or to open eyes for a period of at least six hours after injury. In their series, fewer mass lesions occurred than in adults with injuries of comparable severity (Becker et al., 1977; Jennett et al., 1977). Intracerebral hematomas were rare in the pediatric patient. However, marked diffuse cerebral swelling on serial CT scans, with obliteration of the ventricles and cisterns (Figure 10-1A), followed by enlargement of the ventricles to normal size (or larger), over time (Figure 10-1B) was found in one-third of the cases. In view of the low mortality in this series, the severity of the neurologic deficits reported was remarkable. Oculovestibular function was impaired or absent in 30% of the patients, nearly one-third had bilaterally fixed pupils at the time of admission, and one-third exhibited extension to pain or flaccidity. These findings led Bruce and colleagues to infer that closed head injury in children results primarily in diffuse injury to the white matter. They suggested that the cerebral swelling reflects cerebrovascular congestion resulting in greater blood volume and ultimately impairing intracranial response to changes in pressure.

From the grave neurologic condition and relatively favorable prognosis for

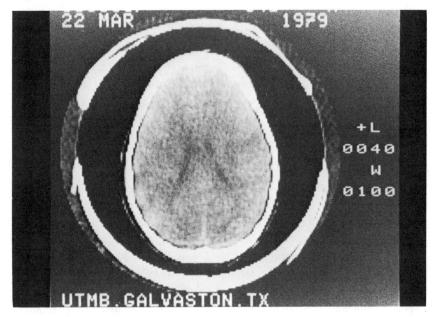

Fig. 10-1. Computerized tomographic scans obtained on the day of severe head injury (22 March 1979) and three months later (31 May 1979) in an eight-year-old boy. Initial Glasgow Coma Scale score was 7; he was unable to follow simple commands for 40 days postinjury. Figure 10-1A (above) shows initial cerebral swelling, reflected by the obliterated lateral ventricles that subsequently enlarged (Fig. 10-1B; below).

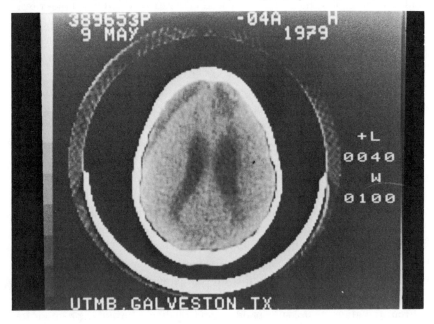

survival in their series, Bruce and his coworkers (1978) concluded that "if the threshold for neurophysiological dysfunction is lower in children than in adults, then for the same input force to the brain, the recorded neurological picture will be worse in the child." The authors also noted that their findings indicated a lower mortality rate than in previous studies of children with severe injury (Gruszkiewicz, Doron, and Peyser, 1973; Hendrick et al., 1964). Hendrick, Harwood-Nash, and Hudson (1964) found that "decerebrate" coma was associated with a 44% mortality. Whether this variation in outcome reflects differences in case selection and referral pattern or is related to intracranial pressure monitoring and aggressive treatment of raised intracranial pressure in the patients remains unclear.

An exception to the rare finding of mass lesions in pediatric closed head injury is brain injury occurring at birth or in the early postnatal period. Acute subdural hematoma was found in 25% of perinatal brain injuries described by Natelson and Sayers (1973). Depressed skull fracture was also a common complication of birth injury.

The acute manifestations of mild, as well as severe closed head injury may differ in children and adults. Hendrick et al. (1964) reported that in 86% of the pediatric admissions, the patients were conscious when initially examined in the emergency room. Their mental status was often characterized by drowsiness, confusion, and irritability. Anterograde and retrograde amnesia were reported by Klonoff and Low (1974) to be less frequent in pediatric closed head injury patients under nine years old than in older children. However, ambiguities in evaluating the presence of amnesia in young children may have influenced the results.

Delayed impairment of consciousness within three hours after a lucid interval in children with apparently mild closed head injury has been described by Todorow and Heiss (1978). In their series of 300 consecutive admissions (age 4 to 14 years), they found that secondary disturbance of consciousness occurred in 24 cases (8%). They described this state as a "fall asleep syndrome," from the German "Einschlafsyndrom," a term introduced by Lange-Cosack and Tepfer (1973).

From the clinical description by Todorow and Heiss, it would appear that the most easily elicted motor response during the period of delayed impairment of consciousness was localizing to painful stimuli. Incomprehensible speech was mentioned, although the degree of eye opening to stimulation was unclear from their study. Neurologic signs, including pupillary changes, were present in nearly one-half the children during the period of impaired consciousness. In contrast to the frequent involvement of intracranial hematoma or other major complications associated with delayed disturbance of consciousness in head-injured adults, the authors reported that the level of consciousness progressively improved within five hours after onset in all the children studied; neurologic findings were completely normal by the second day after injury. The EEG findings during the period of neurologic deterioration were not reported, nor were CT scans described. It is plausible to suggest that this state may reflect a transient phase of cerebral swelling that might be evidenced by compressed ventricles and cisterns on the CT scan.

A clinical picture of delayed impairment of consciousness and neurologic deficit is associated with convulsions after apparently mild head injury in children under 10 years of age (Oka, Kaka, Matsushima, and Ando, 1977; Takahashi and Nakazawa, 1980). The latent period prior to deterioration in level of consciousness ranges from a few minutes to six hours, whereas Takahashi and Nakazawa (1980) reported a variable period of recovery that extended to 47 days. In the EEG, generalized slowing was predominant in all patients studied by Takahashi and Nakazawa (1980). The authors in both studies postulated that delayed neurologic deterioration after apparently mild head injury in children may represent a syndrome of "traumatic spreading depression." Evidence from experiments with animals suggests that a weak faradic or mechanical stimulus to the exposed cortex may induce a persistent reduction of cortical electrical activity that spreads to other cortical regions and results in the development of epileptic discharges. This possibility awaits confirmation by more definitive electrophysiologic studies after mild head injury in children.

Neuropsychological sequelae

Bruce, Schut, Bruno, Wood, and Sutton (1978) have reported that 90% of a series of pediatric closed head injury patients showed a good recovery or only moderate disability after an injury that produced coma (Glasgow Scale score of 8 or less) and pervasive neurologic deficit. Although the focus of their study was on the pathophysiology and clinical management of acute closed head injury in children, they convey the impression of relatively minor residual deficit after severe injury. Brink, Imbus, and Woo-Sam (1980) reported followup data on physical and cognitive recovery one year after injury in 344 children and adolescents who had been comatose at least 24 hours. Consistent with their previous results, the authors noted that less than 10% of the series had normal neurologic findings and that cognitive function remained impaired in about two-thirds of those cases. In contrast, nearly three-fourths of the total sample recovered ambulation and were capable of self-care.

This disparity in outcome findings suggests that observations of improved motor function and adjustment to activities of daily living in children who have sustained severe head injury may lead one to overestimate the quality of cognitive recovery. A review of research on neuropsychological recovery from closed head injury in children shows, however, that cognitive impairment frequently persists after severe injury despite the disappearance of focal motor and sensory deficits and the resumption of daily activities. The resultant behavioral changes may be classified according to their time-course. "Early" effects appear after termination of coma, whereas "late" effects are manifested after resolution of confusion and may involve relatively permanent changes. Although previous studies have suggested that grossly aberrant behavior is frequently transient and confined to the initial phase of recovery, the contention that "significant sequelae" are rare is contrary to the evidence.

Early behavioral effects

During the initial phase of recovery, children exhibit signs of confusion, disorientation, and possibly paramnesia that closely resemble the manifestations described after closed head injury in adults (Chapter 4). The transition from coma to normal orientation may be accompanied by anterograde (posttraumatic) and retrograde amnesia, lethargy, and akinesia (Klonoff and Low, 1974, Todorow, 1975). Amnesia in young children is difficult to measure; age-based norms for temporal orientation are unavailable. Heightened irritability, drowsiness, and confusion may dominate the mental status in children who remain conscious (Hendrick et al., 1964). Todorow described a "sleeping beauty syndrome" characterized by an "akinetic mutistic state" in which the child copes with feelings of helplessness and the restraint imposed by life-support equipment by withdrawing from the environment. The author interpreted the child's effort to remain motionless and apathetic despite signs of neurologic improvement as an attempt to escape a frightening situation.

Blau (1936) described six cases of posttraumatic psychosis in children who required transfer from the neurosurgical service to a psychiatric unit for periods of two to four weeks. The manifestations included acute excitement with impulsiveness and restlessness. The children were noisy and attempted to get out of bed and cried or screamed continuously. The outstanding feature of these cases was a period of unrestrained emotional and motor behavior accompanied by severe anxiety. Posttraumatic amnesia was present in all six children, but they were able to recognize members of their family shortly after regaining consciousness. The posttraumatic psychosis had completely remitted by the time of followup, which was at least six months after injury.

Residual neuropsychological sequelae

Despite the high incidence of closed head injury among children, there have been remarkably few studies of neuropsychological recovery. Generalization of findings across various investigations is complicated by the lack of uniform criteria for grading the neurologic severity of injury. "Severe" closed head injury in children has been inferred from a duration of coma ranging from at least 30 minutes (Klonoff and Paris, 1974; Klonoff, Low, and Clark, 1977) to at least one week (Brink, Garrett, Hale, Woo-Sam, and Nickel, 1970). Richardson (1963) defined severe injury on the basis of a posttraumatic amnesia that exceeded seven days. The studies have also differed with respect to the definition of coma. Methodologic problems have arisen from the wide range of assessment techniques. Several studies are limited to the reporting of overall intellectual level (cf. Brink et al., 1970). Specific testing of learning and memory has been less often performed (Fuld and Fisher, 1977; Levin and Eisenberg, 1979 a,b). In view of the claim that children recover more readily than adults after closed head injury, the time-course of study becomes a major consideration. Consequently, serial testing of children (Klonoff and Clark, 1977; Klonoff and Low, 1974) or at least evaluation after an extended interval (Brink et al., 1979; Richardson, 1963) are essential to evaluate the long-range implications of findings during earlier stages of recovery. Our review of the late neuropsychological effects of closed head injury is organized according to the function investigated.

Language   Hécaen (1976) described 26 cases of acquired aphasia in children, including 16 cases of head trauma, who ranged in age from six to 16 years and who were studied over varying periods. Although these closed head injury patients included four children considered to have primary right hemisphere damage, bilateral injury could not be excluded in these cases. Aphasic disturbance was characterized by a period of mutism, which persisted for as long as three months, reduced initiation of speech, and the absence of paraphasias. Anomia was frequently present during the acute period and tended to persist, whereas impairment of auditory comprehension was uncommon and showed rapid improvement. Alexia also resolved within a brief period, but disturbance of writing was more prolonged. Acalculia was a frequent concomitant. Hécaen concluded that acquired aphasia has a better prognosis in children than in adults.

    Levin and Eisenberg (1979b) evaluated language deficit after closed head injury by giving the Neurosensory Center Comprehensive Examination for Aphasia (Spreen and Benton, 1969) to 64 children and adolescents following resolution of posttraumatic confusion. Language deficit was present during the first six months after injury in nearly one-third of the series. Similar to the pattern of aphasic defects found in adults after closed head injury, anomia was the most common deficit and impairment of repetition was rare. Comprehension of oral language was impaired in only 11% of the patients. Followup examinations showed impressive recovery in young children, whereas residual deficits persisted when patients were injured during late adolescence. Closed head injury associated with focal left hemisphere injury (e.g., hematoma) was compatible with either full recovery or relatively isolated residual defects, such as anomia or deficient word retrieval.

Residual impairment of oral expression, reflected by a reduction in spontaneous speech, was reported by Gaidolfi and Vignolo (1980) in four of 21 patients when they were examined nearly ten years after they had sustained a closed head injury that produced coma.

Memory   Relatively few studies have assessed the capacity of head-injured children to store and retrieve new information. Richardson (1963) tested ten closed head injury patients (five to 18 years' old) with "very severe concussion" who had been in coma more than seven days and were examined at least 18 months after injury. Results based on selected items of the Stanford-Binet and the Benton Visual Retention Tests disclosed memory deficit in all the patients, despite improvement in fine motor skills and in adjustment to daily activities. The importance of assessing long-term storage and retrieval was also demonstrated by Fuld and Fisher (1977), who serially studied two pediatric closed head injury patients and administered the selective reminding test (Buschke and Fuld, 1974). Consistent with Richardson's results, the authors found that the recovery of long-term memory lagged behind the resolution of motor deficit.

Levin and Eisenberg (1979 a,b) and Levin and Grossman (1976) employed a modified version of the selective reminding test and a continuous recognition memory test to evaluate residual memory deficit in children and adolescents after clearing of posttraumatic amnesia. The findings indicate that long-term storage and retrieval, as measured by the selective reminding test, were particularly affected; nearly one-half the patients with closed head injuries of varying severity had an impairment of memory, which was inferred from scores that fell below the fourth percentile of control subjects of comparable age. Figure 10-2 indicates that closed head injuries that produced coma (unresponsiveness to commands) for periods of 24 hours or more (Grade II, III), resulted in greater impairment of consistent retrieval from long-term storage than mild injury that caused only momentary or no loss of consciousness and no neurologic deficit.

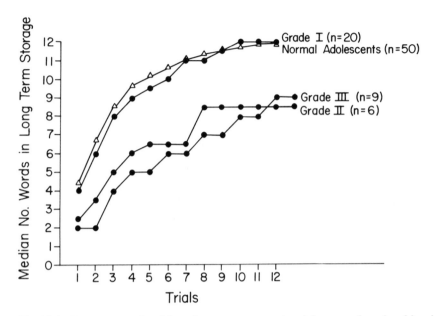

Fig. 10-2. Consistent retrieval from long-term storage in adolescents after closed head injury of varying severity. Grade I, momentary or no loss of consciousness; Grade II, coma duration up to 24 hours; Grade III, coma duration exceeding 24 hours. [From Levin, H.S., and Eisenberg, H.M. (1979a). Neuropsychological outcome of closed head injury in children and adolescents. *Child's Brain*, 5:281–292. Reproduced with permission of the publisher.]

Impaired capacity for incrementing the amount of information acquired across trials is shown in Figure 10-2 by the divergent memory functions. Levin and Eisenberg (1979 a,b) also found that the proportion of patients with residual memory deficit increased according to the severity of acute injury as measured by the Glasgow Coma Scale. An excessively high number of false positive errors characterized the continuous recognition memory of severely injured children and adolescents, a pattern similar to that found in young adults after closed head injury (Hannay, Levin, and Grossman, 1979).

The longitudinal recovery of memory after closed head injury in children remains largely unexplored. As noted, Gaidolfi and Vignolo (1980) reported evidence of a verbal memory deficit nearly ten years later in nearly one-quarter of children who had sustained a closed head injury that produced coma. Memory span for spatial location was less frequently impaired. Our own experience suggests that memory deficit may persist and interfere with progress in school, despite recovery of normal intelligence.

Intellectual ability and school achievement   School failure, transfer to a special education program, and referral to resource teachers for remediation in specific areas have been documented in followup studies of children with closed head injury (Brink et al., 1970; Fuld and Fisher, 1977; Heiskanen and Kaste, 1974; Klonoff and Clark, 1977). The poor academic progress is related to such neurologic deficits as ataxia and aphasia, as well as to neuropsychological sequelae (Brink et al., 1970; Klonoff and Clark, 1977; Klonoff and Low, 1974). In a longitudinal study of 231 children, the majority of whom sustained mild closed head injury, Klonoff and Clark (1977) found progressive increments in IQ over a five-year period in both children younger and older than nine years at the time of injury. However, intellectual deficit in these patients was demonstrated throughout the course of the study by comparison with a control group of pediatric patients without neurologic disorder. In an earlier study, Klonoff and Low (1974) reported an average decrement of 10 IQ points when evaluation was performed one year after injury.

Marked cognitive impairment has been reported in followup studies of children who had sustained severe closed head injury. Flach and Malmros (1972) found that nearly one-half of 131 patients exhibited cognitive deficit when tested eight to 10 years after injury. Although the descriptive statistics are not presented, it is reported that the Performance IQ was most affected. In a 10-year followup study of 21 pediatric closed head injury patients who had been in coma for varying durations, Gaidolfi and Vignolo (1980) found that four cases had WAIS IQ scores below 80.

The most discouraging long-term findings after severe closed head injury have been reported by Brink, Garrett, Hale, Woo-Sam, and Nickel (1970) in their study of 52 patients (age range two to 18 years at injury) who were comatose for at least one week (median duration four weeks) and tested on the WISC or Stanford-Binet one to seven years after injury. In contrast to the eventual resumption of activities of daily living and ambulation in nearly all patients, testing disclosed that only one-third of the children had an IQ within one standard deviation of the population mean (i.e., an IQ of at least 85). Thirty-seven percent of the group showed severe cognitive impairment, as reflected by an IQ below 70. A direct relationship between coma duration and residual IQ with greater impairment in children who were under eight years old at the time of injury was found. Figure 10-3 shows that there was a greater decrement in IQ as a function of coma duration in young children, whereas the slope of the

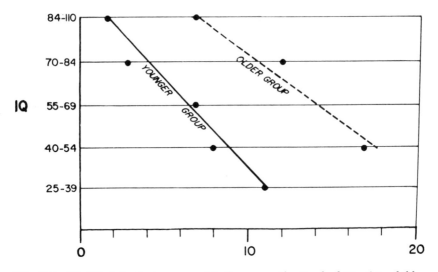

Fig. 10-3. IQ (Wechsler Scale appropriate for age or the Stanford-Binet) in children who sustained severe closed head injury (coma duration of at least one week) plotted against duration of coma. The coma durations of children in each IQ category (corresponding to 1 S.D. from the population mean) are averaged. [From Brink, J.D. et al. (1970). Recovery of motor and intellectual function in children sustaining severe head injuries. *Dev. Med. Child Neurol. 12:*565–571. Reproduced with permission of the authors and publisher.]

function is less for patients who were over ten years old at the time of injury. Although the sample of pediatric closed head injury patients studied by Brink, Garrett, Hale, Woo-Sam, and Nickel (1970) was drawn from a rehabilitation hospital and presumably excluded children who had made a good recovery from severe closed head injury, there are no published reports indicating sparing of cognitive function in children who have sustained closed head injuries of similar severity.

The greater vulnerability of infants and toddlers to long-term cognitive impairment (four to 14 years after severe closed head injury), as compared to preschool- and kindergarten-aged children, was recently confirmed in a follow-up study of 50 patients treated on the neurosurgical service at the Klinikum, West Berlin (Lange-Cosack et al., 1979). Duration of coma was directly related to the extent of residual deficit. The presence of acute brain injury was frequently substantiated by CT findings, and serial CT scans disclosed evidence of ventricular dilation in several cases. The authors concluded that their results corroborated the findings of Brink, Garrett, Hale, Woo-Sam, and Nickel (1970), who administered the WISC to ten severely head-injured children (minimum posttraumatic amnesia seven days, median coma duration 28 days) at intervals ranging from 1.5 to 13.5 years after injury. Richardson (1963) found that the IQ of the patients ranged from borderline defective to low average. Preinjury data indicating that nine of the patients had previously functioned at the average level or better led the authors to estimate that there had been a decrement of 10 to 30 IQ points. Levin and Eisenberg (1979b) obtained preinjury achievement and IQ scores and found that the WISC-R administered at least six months after injury has generally shown a decline in cognitive ability.

In summary, the evidence offers no support for the view that children are spared residual cognitive deficit after severe closed head injury. Although there has been no systematic investigation that included Glasgow Coma Scale scoring, CT findings, and analysis of premorbid factors in relation to cognitive recovery, the data suggest greater vulnerability of young children (less than nine years of age) to the neuropsychological effects of head injury as compared to older children.

Related neuropsychological sequelae   Neuropsychological assessment has been generally limited to standardized measurement of intellectual ability in studies of recovery from closed head injury in children. Klonoff and his colleagues (Klonoff, Low, and Clark, 1977; Klonoff and Low, 1974) administered a comprehensive series of tests that included techniques developed by Reitan, Benton, and Kløve to 231 pediatric cases in whom mild closed head injuries predominated. Initial and one-year followup findings disclosed that slow visuomotor performance on the Trailmaking Test, reduced finger and foot tapping speed, impaired formboard assembly, and defective maze performance were among the most marked deficits when closed head injury patients were compared to neurologically intact children of similar demographic background. Levin and Eisenberg (1979 a,b) found visuospatial deficit, as measured by construction of block designs using three-dimensional models (Benton and Fogel, 1962) and by copying the Bender designs, occurred in nearly one-third of these pediatric patients tested after resolution of posttraumatic amnesia. The likelihood of visuospatial impairment was directly related to the duration of coma and to the severity of acute injury as reflected by ratings on the Glasgow Coma Scale at the time of admission. Consistent with the finding of slow motor speed reported by Klonoff and Low, reaction time was frequently found to be prolonged after closed head injury in adolescents and thumb-finger opposition was slow in head-injured children (six to 11 years). Diminished somatosensory performance on tests of stereognosis, finger localization, and graphesthesia was present in about one-fourth of the total series. Information about the persistence of these sequelae awaits further progress of this longitudinal study. It may be inferred, however, that the range of neuropsychological deficits during the first six months after closed head injury in children resembles that found in adults.

Social and psychiatric effects of closed head injury in children

Studies of the quality of recovery from closed head injury in children have generally considered social adjustment, although there has been wide variation in assessment techniques. Descriptive information obtained during the course of a neurologic and/or a psychiatric examination has been common to most studies. Data based on a standardized interview of patients and their parents, however, have been less often obtained. Consequently, disparities in the presence of behavioral sequelae may reflect procedural differences. Disagreement stems primarily from variation in the type of behavioral problems and inferences regarding their etiology. There is greater agreement in the literature concerning the occurrence of emotional maladjustment in head-injured children.

It has been shown that head injury producing persistent coma and acute neurologic deficit frequently results in residual behavioral changes. In a study of 23 predominantly preschool-aged closed head injury patients who had been comatose for 24 hours or more, Hjern and Nylander (1964) found that severe psychiatric sequelae were present at least six months after injury in five patients and were accompanied by neurologic deficit in all these cases. The characteristics of the behavioral disorder were not described in detail. Children in coma at least one week were examined one to seven years later and found by Brink, Garrett, Hale, Woo-Sam, and Nickel (1970) to exhibit persistent behavioral changes that varied according to age and injury; children who were under ten years of age at the time of injury exhibited hyperactivity, short attention span, impulsiveness, and aggressive behavior, whereas children who were at least ten years old at the time of injury manifested poor judgment and affective disturbance.

A followup assessment by Flach and Malmros (1972), eight to ten years after closed head injury of varying severity, found that 27% of their patients were "socially maladjusted." Severe complications of acute injury, such as cardiac arrest and respiratory failure, were related to chronic social problems in this study. The authors depicted a characteristic "slowness" in mental function and motor behavior, but were unable to confirm the observations of hyperkinesis reported by Brink et al. Ten children and adolescents who had periods of post-traumatic amnesia for at least a week were subsequently found by Richardson (1963) to require a "sheltered and tolerant environment" and to frequently manifest perseverative behavior associated with increased anxiety, irritability, and excessive fatigability. The findings of these relatively recent studies resemble Blau's 1936 description of the "posttraumatic psychopathic personality" in which the cardinal characteristics were overactivity, restlessness, destructiveness, aggression, temper tantrums, and delinquency. From serial observations, Blau inferred that behavioral disorder attributable to brain injury became progressively apparent after convalescence from the acute injury when the patient engaged in socially unacceptable behavior that brought him into conflict with the community.

Behavioral sequelae one to two years after closed head injury were systematically evaluated by Klonoff and Paris (1974) on the basis of behavioral observations and parental interviews. Preinjury learning disabilities and other "developmental anomalies" were common in boys, particularly those in the under–nine-year-old age group. Males were also found to be more vulnerable to developing behavioral disturbance after closed head injury; increased irritability was commonly observed in young boys at both the one- and two-year post-injury examinations, whereas "personality changes" were frequently reported in both sexes irrespective of age. Overall, slightly more than one-half of the total series (n 231) evidenced at least one residual behavioral problem two years after injury. Notwithstanding the alleged rare occurrence of the "posttraumatic syndrome" in children (Jennett, 1972), 29% of the children studied by Klonoff and Low complained of headache during the first year and 18% continued to complain of headache during the second year after injury. Dizziness (vertigo, giddiness) was common in boys during the first year after injury, but greatly diminished in frequency thereafter. Deterioration in the child's relationships was primarily found in the home, affecting about 10% in the children during the first year and 5% of the patients during the second postinjury year. Psychological reactions to head trauma were predominated by denial (about two-thirds to three-fourths of the patients depending on age and sex) and greater caution in response to potential dangers. Parents frequently reported that they became increasingly anxious and apprehensive concerning the possibility of residual brain damage in their children; there was also a trend toward greater parental protectiveness. Although behavioral sequelae were pervasive in the children studied by Klonoff and Low, it is difficult to ascertain from their findings the proportion of children with major alterations of behavior.

Several studies have analyzed the potentially moderating effects of age, severity and locus of injury, premorbid factors, and social conditions on the emergence of behavioral disturbance after closed head injury. In a comprehensive analysis of age effects, Klonoff and Low (1974) found no difference in the relative frequency of sequelae and only minor variation in the rank order of problems when children who were under nine years of age at the time of injury were compared to the older patients. Similarly, Shaffer et al. (1975) reported that age had no bearing on the occurrence of behavioral problems resulting from closed head injury with unilateral depressed skull fracture. The authors reported that the severity of the injury, as measured by duration of coma, was related to the likelihood of later psychiatric disturbance, whereas the side of depressed skull fracture was inconsequential. These findings were confirmed by Naughton (1971), who reported no variation in the behavioral disturbance resulting from closed head injury associated with left versus right hemispheric injury, whereas involvement of the brain stem had adverse prognostic implications.

The nature of the etiologic factors in the behavioral disorders of children after closed head injury has been a subject of debate. The view that premorbid disturbance primarily contributes to posttraumatic behavioral disorder is reflected in Jennett's contention that relatively few head-injured children "have behavioral disorders, and many who do so prove to have been psychosocially maladjusted before the injury." Extensive clinical observations of head-injured children transferred to psychiatric units led Blau (1936) to reach the opposite conclusion in that he stressed the role of brain injury in dramatically altering the character of children and likened the effects to postencephalitic personality changes.

Partial support for both views was provided by Black, Blumer, Wellner, and Walker (1971), who found that behavioral problems antedated the occurrence of closed head injury in one-third of their patients. Contrary to Jennett's conclusion, however, the authors found that one-fifth of the previously disturbed children developed behavioral symptoms after injury that were unlike the problems manifested before injury. Moreover, posttraumatic behavioral disturbance was observed with similar frequency in children who had no previous history of emotional maladjustment. From their five-year longitudinal study of long-term sequelae, Black and his associates concluded that "although premorbid personality may influence the nature of posttraumatic sequelae, the injury itself appears to be responsible for the development of problems." They viewed the relative contributions of brain injury vs. the child's psychological reaction to trauma in producing behavioral disturbance as an unresolved question.

Summary

Investigations of outcome after closed head injury in children have increasingly employed neurologic indices of acute injury severity, serial or long-term follow-up examinations, and neuropsychological methods of assessment. Although confident prediction of the level of neuropsychological recovery from closed head injury of varying severity in children of differing ages awaits further study, the previously held view that children are relatively impervious to cognitive impairment after such injury is clearly not supported by the available data. Several studies have documented persistent, marked cognitive impairment concomitant with a decline in school achievement after severe head injury in children. The effects of primary brain damage of the immediate impact type and secondary brain injury associated with late complications (e.g., hypoxia, metabolic disturbance) must be differentiated to elucidate the relationship between mechanisms of injury and neuropsychological sequelae.

Studies to date suggest that memory and motor skill are the most seriously impaired functions after closed head injury in children. In contrast, language development is relatively resistant to the effects of closed head injury as reflected by predominantly mild aphasic defects and their remarkable reversibility. Behavioral disturbance has been demonstrated to occur after severe closed head injury in children, although a consensus has not been reached concerning the most salient features of postinjury personality changes. The relative contributions of brain damage, preinjury characteristics, and the postinjury social milieu to behavioral disturbance remain obscure.

11. Rehabilitation

The remarkable increase in the rate of survival from severe head injury during the past two decades means that there is (and will continue to be) a steadily increasing number of posttraumatic patients with significant behavioral deficits who must be helped to attain a satisfactory life adjustment. Consequently, the provision of adequate rehabilitative services for these brain-damaged survivors is of major importance. In this connection, Jennett (1975) has pointed out that "the tremendous efforts expended on intensive treatment in the early weeks after injury are often largely wasted by the failure to provide the means whereby the full potential for recovery can be achieved during the later stages," and he has called attention to the burden placed on available rehabilitative services by patients with residual cognitive impairment and behavioral disturbance. However, as will be seen, few studies have attempted to assess the effects of rehabilitation on neuropsychological recovery from severe closed head injury. Research on outcome and the efficiency of rehabilitation is complicated by heterogeneity in type and severity of the injury; variation in selection criteria; individual differences in preinjury ability; and difficulty in carrying out a controlled study because head-injured patients not enrolled in a rehabilitation program also must be identified and followed (Field, 1976).

Rehabilitation after severe closed head injury

Experiences with severe head injury gained during World War II led to a shift in strategy from advocating prolonged bedrest to prescribing physical therapy and cognitive stimulation at the earliest feasible time (Höök, 1969; Maury et al., 1970). This approach was advocated in order to prevent complications (e.g., orthostatic arterial hypotension) that result from prolonged inactivity. Höök contended that an excessively long period of bedrest contributes to the development of such "postconcussional" symptoms as headache and fatigue. Although the availability of facilities and the pressure for beds in acute care hospitals frequently determine the length of time between initial recovery from head injury and transfer to a rehabilitation unit, the evidence to date suggests that therapeutic treatment is most effective if it is initiated at the earliest opportunity during the first six months of convalescence (Bond and Brooks, 1976). It has been suggested that a critical period may exist during which rehabilitation produces gains in excess of the natural course of recovery and the importance of involving the family is also emphasized. Counseling the family during the early phase of recovery to prepare it for possible changes in the patient's behavior may help to avert inappropriate reactions that complicate rehabilitative efforts (Thomsen, 1974).

Serial observations of families during the subacute stage of the patient's recovery indicate that denial of disability or misinterpretation of the patient's condition are common reactions (Romano, 1974; Rosin, 1977). Denial may be expressed in the form of the "sleeping beauty" myth that a deeply comatose patient will rapidly recover as if awaking from normal sleep. It may also take the form of "seeing" an improvement in motor functioning that in fact has not occurred. Unresolved denial by the family may lead to unrealistic expectations and an inability to set limits on the patient's behavior after discharge from the hospital. In the absence of counseling prior to the discharge of the patient from the acute care center, the family may pressure the patient to resume responsibilities prematurely and thus expose him to painful frustrating experiences. Maladaptive responses by members of the family may also include anger toward the professional staff expressed by uncooperativeness or misinterpretation of information, with the subsequent contention that they were not adequately informed.

The typical rehabilitation team for patients with severe head injury consists of a psychiatrist, a physical therapist, a speech therapist, an occupational therapist, and a psychologist. Consultants from neurosurgery and psychiatry and social workers and teachers are also frequently involved in rehabilitation programs. Detailed description of the various types of therapy are provided by Goldstein (1980) and Renfrew (1971). Specific approaches to rehabilitation may be characterized with respect to selection of patients, goals, aspects of the treatment program, and involvement of the patient's family.

   The most detailed description of a rehabilitation program specifically designed for head injury that has been published in recent years is that of the Lowenstein Rehabilitation Hospital in Raanana, Israel (Najenson et al., 1974, 1975; Rosenbaum et al., 1978). According to the authors, active management may begin while the patient is still unconscious (cf. Najenson et al., 1974). Passive movement of the joints and mobilization may be carried out to prevent limb contractures and the patient may be exercised on a tilting board to stimulate postural reflexes. Functional movements are encouraged by the physical therapist as the patient becomes better able to cooperate. During the transition from coma to normal orientation, severe behavioral disturbance may emerge; these include agitation, restlessness, and possibly a transient psychosis (see Chapter 9). Behavioral management is facilitated by providing a supportive, calm environment and encouraging the participation of the patient's family in achieving a sense of security and reorientation. On neurosurgical acute care units, administration of a major tranquilizer may be necessary to prevent self-injury in patients who are psychotic and markedly agitated.

   Closed head injury patients and cases with penetrating missile wounds are also accepted in the Lowenstein Program after a longer interval, provided that they have a potential for retraining as reflected by a WAIS Verbal or Performance IQ of at least 80. The program for patients who have emerged from the posttraumatic amnesia phase of recovery begins with comprehensive assessment based on psychological testing, interviews with the family, and behavioral observations of the patient during a trial stay on the unit. From this data base, the staff rates the patient on the five problem areas shown in Table 11-1. Rosenbaum et al. (1978) report that behavioral and environmental problems were the greatest obstacles to recovery in the 13 patients described in their paper.

   The first goal of the treatment program (Table 11-1) is to help the patient develop skills that are indirectly related to holding a job, such as maintaining a positive attitude, improving self-esteem, and increasing cognitive efficiency. The treatment modalities include individual psychotherapy (three to five times weekly) to assist the patient in accepting the consequences of his disability and pursuing activities that emphasize abilities spared by the injury. Acquisition of adaptive behavior is stressed (e.g., requesting assistance at appropriate times) as is psychotherapy for personal problems, including marital conflict and sexual difficulties. The psychotherapist assumes primary responsibility for the design of the patient's rehabilitation program, and the therapist–patient relationship may be used to encourage participation in a wide range of activities. Cognitive retraining consists of speech therapy, remedial reading, writing, arithmetic, and a graded series of perceptual motor tasks. The authors found little evidence of

Table 11-1. Problem areas rated at the time of initial assessment at the Lowenstein Rehabilitation Hospital°

Cognitive deficit	*Motor control*
1. Speech/language	1. Eye–hand incoordination
2. Perception	2. Slowness
3. Memory	3. Nonfunctional limbs
a. Short term	
b. Long term	
Behavioral problems	*"Neurotic" symptoms*
1. Irresponsible behavior	1. Depression
2. Socially inappropriate behavior	2. Anxiety
3. Exhibitionistic behavior	3. Low self-esteem
Environmental problems	
1. Rejecting spouse	
2. Lack of social support	
3. Financial support	

°From Rosenbaum, M. (1978) *Scand. J. Rehab. Med.* 10:1–6. Reproduced with permission of the author and publisher.

generalization from training on specific cognitive tasks to other activities and thus recommended the use of such devices as a calculator and typewriter to compensate for severe residual deficit in modes of response (e.g., writing) or cognitive processes (e.g., calculation).

Vocational rehabilitation in the Lowenstein program begins with assignment to a workshop in which simple assembly tasks designed to assess potential for further instruction are assigned, along with training in work habits and perceptual motor skills (Table 11-1). Production and appropriate work behaviors are rewarded with tokens that can be exchanged by the patient for money in a "bank," which is part of the program. Patients who graduate from a workshop are assigned more demanding jobs within the hospital (e.g., maintenance) or within the rehabilitation workshop. Supervision by the patient's primary therapist is maintained throughout the vocational training. Gradually the patients are placed in semi-sheltered jobs in the community.

Group activities are designed to develop a therapeutic milieu and social support. The staff attempt to generalize gains observed in the program to the community by engaging the participation of the family and the employer. Families are seen in group therapy in an effort to facilitate understanding and acceptance of the patient's disabilities and alterations in personality. Goals of family therapy include discussing realistic expectations regarding the patient's behavior, and discouraging over-protective behavior by assisting family members in examining their guilt feelings. The rehabilitation team also acts as the patient's advocate in negotiating financial compensation from the government, particularly with respect to brain injury sustained by soldiers during combat.

Outcome of rehabilitation after severe closed head injury

Few authors have systematically studied the variables that influence the course and effectiveness of rehabilitation after closed head injury. In view of the numerous variables that potentially affect the outcome of rehabilitation and the difficulty in studying any single factor in isolation, the available findings should be interpreted cautiously. Field (1976) has emphasized the constraints imposed on research in this area by nonuniform criteria for assessing recovery in rehabilitation centers and heterogeneity in the injuries that typically diminish the size of well-defined groups (e.g., a series of cases with left hemisphere mass lesion). Difficulty in obtaining a nonrehabilitated group with head injury of severity comparable to treated patients also complicates research. Notwithstanding these issues, Field concludes that the available evidence supports the effectiveness of rehabilitation.

The outcome of rehabilitation in patients rendered initially vegetative or severely disabled by head injury was studied by Najenson et al. (1974) in admissions (two-thirds closed head injury patients, one-third missile wound patients) to the Lowenstein Rehabilitation Program. As Table 11-2 indicates, over 15% had died or were still vegetative at the time of discharge from the hospital. Although it is unclear from the table whether the category of "simple work" includes jobs equivalent to positions held prior to injury, it is evident that

Table 11-2. State on discharge of 169 patients and duration of hospital stay[*]

Average stay (months)	No. of patients	State on discharge
1.6	9	Died
5.0	18	Vegetative
6.6	32	Independent in activities of daily living
6.1	36	Capable of sheltered work
4.6	51	Capable of simple work
3.6	23	Capable of professional work
Total Series 5.1	169	

[*]From Najenson, T., Mendelson, L., Schechter, I., David, C., Mintz, N., and Grosswasser, Z. (1974) *Scand. J. Rehab. Med.* 6:5–14. Reproduced with permission of the authors and publisher.

only a small proportion of these patients fully resumed occupational activities after discharge. Followup examination after an undefined interval from the date of discharge disclosed further improvement in two-thirds of the patients who were able to resume work or at least were independent when they left the rehabilitation hospital. Of the 149 patients who participated in the followup assessment, 33 (22%) were found to be capable of working. Again, there was no detailed information concerning the proportion of patients working full-time or the comparability of their employment to their preinjury occupation.

Rosin (1978) has reported on the outcome of rehabilitation for a series of 23 patients with severe brain damage, including 15 closed head injury cases. The patients were referred to the rehabilitation program at the Harzfeld Hospital in Cedera, Israel within a year of injury; 19 patients were considered to be vegetative when they entered the program and four cases were severely disabled. The subsequent course over a three-year period was characterized by a 50% mortality arising from complications including sepsis and pneumonia. Only two patients (9%) of the original series improved to a level of moderate disability. Table 11-3 depicts the neurologic functions that improved during the course of rehabilitation. It will be seen that the most frequent changes were in posture and movement, there being gradual improvement in these functions over a three-year period. Communication within the social environment was also facilitated, although it is likely that severe residual impairment of language was present in many patients because only two were considered by the author to have achieved the level of moderate disability. Patients who were vegetative at six months usually remained in this condition, but a few cases slowly passed through a vegetative state and eventually reached a level of functioning, limited primarily by the focal hemispheric injury.

A recent study by Gilchrist and Wilkinson (1979) investigated the variables relevant to global outcome and return to work after rehabilitation in closed head injury patients under 40 years old who were transferred to a rehabilitation unit in England after periods of coma of at least 24 hours. It was found that the duration of coma and the stability of the patient's family were most closely related to the degree of recovery and the resumption of work. Age was not predictive of outcome in this study of young adults.

In a major study of vocational recovery after head injury, Dresser et al. (1973) obtained long-term followup information on 864 veterans who had sustained a head injury during the Korean Campaign. Closed head injury accounted for about one-fourth of the total series. Although the followup interviews were arranged by the American National Red Cross and the study was not specifically done within a rehabilitation context, it is likely that many participants in

Table 11-3. Changes in neurologic status over a one-year period°

	Group A (n 17)	Group B (n 6)
Swallowing improved	4	1
Muscle tone		
Increase	4	2
Decrease	3	—
Increase and decrease	3	
Tremor		
Appearance	1	1
Disappearance	1	
Posture improved	6	2
Movement improved	7	3
Speech		
Improved	2	3
Sounds	3	1
Meaningful contact	4 (+ ?1)	
Already in contact	1	2
Confusion improved	2	3
Behaviour improved	—	3

From Rosin, A.J. (1978) *Scand. J. Rehab. Med. 10*:33–38. Reproduced with permission of the author and publisher.
° *Group A*, patients in whom meaningful communication could not be initially established because of incomplete consciousness.
Group B, patients who exhibited additional problems, particularly behavioral disturbance.

the study had had extended care in military or Veterans Administration hospitals. Interviews completed 15 years after injury disclosed that gainful employment, i.e., receiving a salary for work, was strongly related to preinjury mental status (measured by the Armed Forces Qualification Test at the time of induction) and preinjury occupational status. The authors noted that these two preinjury characteristics were correlated variables. Employment following injury was less likely in patients in whom injury was complicated by a long duration of coma, the presence of aphasia, motor impairment, or seizures that persisted more than one month after injury. An additive effect when more than two factors were weighted in the same direction (e.g., the combination of low preinjury mental status and motor deficit was associated with a rate of gainful employment of 59 vs. 84% for patients with a high level of preinjury mental status and no motor deficits) was also noted. The prognostic significance of preinjury occupational status in civilians entering a rehabilitation program following severe closed head injury had been reported earlier by Rusk, Block, and Lowman (1969). These studies suggest that preinjury characteristics and neurologic indices of injury severity are the principal determinants of outcome.

In his review of the literature concerning outcome from rehabilitation, Field (1976) commented on the relationship between emotional sequelae of head injury and the gains achieved through rehabilitation. The author observed that patients with diminished self-insight fare worse than those patients with realistic self-appraisal, a finding that awaits further study. Motivational level was also cited by Field as a potent variable as were the reaction to the patient by members of the community and the role of the family in shaping the outcome of rehabilitation. Available evidence suggests that residual cognitive impairment and subsequent support from the family may interact. Research carried out in Glasgow has indicated that posttraumatic cognitive impairment has an adverse impact on family cohesion, whereas the social unit is far more resistant to the patient's physical handicap (Bond and Brooks, 1976). Finally, Field concluded that there is no evidence that patients who apply for compensation or disability benefits are less likely to return to work after severe closed head injury than patients who do not apply for such benefits.

Strategies of rehabilitation may be refined as investigators determine the "training characteristics" (Miller, 1980) of patients with severe head injury, i.e., their capacity to acquire skills and transfer learning across settings. Miller (1980) recently demonstrated that after severely injured patients emerge from prolonged posttraumatic amnesia, they can improve their performance on a series of spatial formboards with extended practice. In extrapolating the findings to rehabilitation, he suggested that breaking a task down into successive steps may be a useful training strategy. This preliminary study underscores the need for further work to find training techniques that can be adjusted according to individual differences and initial impairment.

Relevance of evoked potentials to rehabilitation

Rappaport et al. (1977, 1978) have studied head-injured patients who were transferred after varying intervals to the rehabilitation department of the Santa Clara Medical Center in San Jose, California and who were assessed by visual and auditory evoked cortical potentials. Concurrent with the evoked potential measurement, disability was rated using a modified version of the Glasgow Outcome Scale (Jennett and Bond, 1975), which was expanded to include ratings on adjustment to daily activities, capacity for personal hygiene and feeding, and employability. The revised Glasgow Outcome Scale also incorporates the Glasgow Coma Scale, which is useful in evaluating persistently vegetative or severely disabled patients. This procedure yields a range of total scores (0 to 30) from which the authors derive a classification of outcome using eight categories (a copy of the scale is in the Appendix).

Deviation of major components of the evoked potential from the waveform obtained in normal controls was rated for presence or absence of major peaks, delays in expected latencies, and overall pattern. Composite ratings of abnormalities in the long latency components of the visual- and auditory-evoked potentials had the highest correlation with degree of disability ($r = 0.51$), with slightly lower correlations for long latency responses of each modality considered separately. The relationship between the ratings of short latency components of the auditory-evoked potential and disability was weak. It is generally believed that the long latency components of the evoked potential reflect nonspecific cortical activity, whereas short latency components of the auditory-evoked potential represent activity of the eighth nerve and brain stem nuclei (Starr, 1978). Consequently, the findings by Rappaport and his associates suggest that evoked potential correlates of cortical acitvity may be useful prognostic indicators of rehabilitation. Further research is needed to explore the relationship between neuropsychological findings after closed head injury and specific alterations of evoked potential, particularly with respect to recordings obtained during the performance of cognitive tasks.

Memory therapy

In a prophetic paper concerning rehabilitation after head injury, Lewin (1968) asserted that "if one were to pick out the one symptom which makes rehabilitation difficult, one would select impairment of memory" (p. 467). He also called for the development of techniques to facilitate recovery of memory, a suggestion that has only recently been implemented in systematic studies (cf. Glasgow et al., 1977). Investigation of behavioral strategies to improve memory in normal subjects, however, has a long-established history (Yates, 1966). In a review of the history of mnemonic techniques, Patten (1972) traced the "art of memory" to the sixth century B.C. when orators employed visual imagery of the to-be-remembered material in preparation for speeches. These early practitioners of mnemonics anticipated recent studies by cognitive psychologists that have disclosed that visual imagery often facilitates initial learning and may enhance long-term retention (Paivio, 1971). The finding of facilitation of verbal memory by imagery has been attributed to an additive effect of verbal–semantic coding and imaginal mediation as compared to the typical dependence on the former in retention of verbal material.

On the other hand, task instructions or other manipulations that accentuate the processing of the semantic characteristics of a word (e.g., a query regarding the category of a class to which the noun belongs such as "animal") increase the probability of it being subsequently recalled by normal subjects (cf. Craik and Tulving, 1975). In contrast, instructing the subject to comment about the structural (e.g., is it in upper or lower case letters) or phonemic characteristics (e.g., does it rhyme with the word "white") has no positive effects. Instructions that stress mediation by imagery and conditions that emphasize the semantic encoding of words as they are presented may have in common a "deeper" level of encoding as compared to a more superficial processing of stimuli (Craik and Lockard, 1972). Although the theoretical aspects in which processing of verbal-abstract and nonverbal visual information are incompletely understood, clinical investigations have suggested that utilization of this dual memory encoding system may involve hemispheric functional asymmetry (Milner, 1978). From studies of memory in patients undergoing temporal lobectomy for intractable epilepsy, the hypothesis has been advanced that the left temporal lobe primarily encodes stimuli according to their verbal-semantic characteristics, whereas the right temporal lobe more efficiently processes nonverbal material (Milner, 1978). Consequently, it is possible that the most appropriate mnemonic strategy may vary according to the lateralization of mass lesion and the severity of diffuse injury.

Variations of imagery mnemonics have in common the linking of the to-be-remembered word with some other stimulus that serves as a cue and is also imagined visually. Luria (1968) described the employment of this technique by a professional mnemonist:

> Earlier, if I were to remember the word *America*, I'd have had to stretch a long, long rope across the ocean, from Gorky Street to America, so as not to lose the way. This isn't necessary any more. Say I'm given the word *elephant:* I'd see a zoo. If they gave me *America*, I'd set up an image of Uncle Sam; if *Bismarck*, I'd place my image near the statue of Bismarck; and if I had the word *transcendent*, I'd see my teacher Sherbiny standing and looking at a monument. . . . I don't go through all those complicated operations any more, getting myself to different countries in order to remember words.

Patten (1972) adapted techniques espoused by practitioners of memory training in which a list of items is retained by forming vivid images for each one and associating them in a bizarre manner (e.g., drinking tea from a radio). The second stage of training consists of the learning of a list of "peg" words through visual imagery, followed by experience in learning other lists of items by associating each one with a peg word. Patten found that this technique was effective in facilitating retention by patients with specific impairment of verbal memory resulting from left hemisphere damage. In contrast to their preserved capacity for generating vivid images to compensate for a verbal memory defect, three patients with global memory disorder associated with lesions of the midline structures failed to improve.

Compensation for a specific impairment of verbal memory through use of visual imagery was confirmed by Jones (1974). Immediate and delayed (two hours) recall of pairs of concrete words (e.g., jail–frog) was aided in patients who had undergone a left temporal lobectomy because of intractable epilepsy by showing a fused picture (e.g., a frog in jail) or providing instructions to evoke images for linking words together. No enhancement of memory was found for abstract word pairs (e.g., truth–amount). Visual imagery also facilitated the verbal memory of patients with right temporal lobectomy and normal controls, although the gain was less impressive in these groups. Despite these gains, verbal memory in patients after left temporal lobectomy was still below that in other groups. In agreement with Patten's findings, Jones found that two amnesic patients with bilateral medial temporal lobe damage failed to respond to the imagery technique. Facilitation of verbal memory in patients with left hemisphere cerebral vascular accident was recently reported (Gasparrini and Satz, 1979).

Limitations in the application of imagery training were disclosed in a study of patients in whom cerebral vascular disease predominated (Lewinsohn et al., 1977). Training to link words by bizarre visual imagery improved initial memory performance and 30-minute recall, but no gain was evidenced when the patients were retested one week later. Imagery was less effective in learning to associate names with faces, a source of frustration to many head-injured patients.

Training in imagery mnemonics in patients with closed head injury has been recently studied, primarily in case reports (Table 11-4). Although offering a modest degree of encouragement, the findings summarized in Table 11-4 indicate considerable individual differences in response. Plausible linking imagery may be more appropriate for certain patients than bizarre imagery; self-paced imagery may be more effective than instructions given by the examiner in patients with slowed processing of information. As shown in Table 11-4, mnemonic techniques have been applied primarily to college-educated closed head injury patients. Whether this strategy is appropriate for remediation in head-

Table 11-4. Published studies of memory retraining for head-injured patients

Authors	Subjects (*n*)	Mnemonic technique	Analysis of data	Findings	Comments
Crovitz (1979) USA	Korsakoff (*n* 1), CHI (*n* 1)	Images given by examiner for chaining words. Images were often bizarre. Retrieval cues were also given	Descriptive case report	Free, unassisted recall was unimproved by imagery, but cueing at the time of retrieval was facilitory	Although encouraging, recall was critically dependent on cueing by examiner. No convincing evidence of generalization to daily activities
Crovitz et al. (1979) USA	CHI (*n* 2), HSE. after right temp. lobectomy (*n* 1)	Chaining words through bizarre imagery given by the examiner and self-evoked images; learning to associate word pairs by imagery	Descriptive	Bizarre imagery was helpful in cases where images were given by the examiner, but not when they were self-generated. Plausible images were often preferred to bizarre images. Case 2 (CHI) had enhancement using concrete, plausible images; case 3 performed best with self-paced, concrete images	Individual differences in preference for self-pacing and plausibility of images. Series included two university students. Generalization of findings is questionable
Glasgow et al. (1977) USA	CHI patients (*n* 2)	1. oral rehearsal (case 1) 2. system for asking key questions and rehearsal (case 1) 3. linking visual imagery (case 2) 4. simple visual imagery to associate names with faces	Descriptive	Retention of written material was facilitated in case 1; Face-name pairs were retained better using simple imagery in case 2, whereas complex instructions for linking were ineffective	Both patients were college students with presumably above average preinjury intelligence. Generalization of training was found for case 2 by repeated reference to reminder cards while at home

Abbreviations: CHI, closed head injury; HSE, herpes simplex encephalitis; temp, temporal.

injured patients with less education awaits further investigation. Evidence recently obtained in normal subjects suggests that a high level of intellectual ability may be necessary to employ visual imagery mnemonics to their full advantage (Griffith and Actkinson, 1978).

The assumption that imagery is selectively spared after closed head injury has been questioned by Richardson (1979a) who found that patients with relatively mild closed head injuries exhibited less facilitation than normal subjects in free recall when concrete, rather than abstract nouns were used. When tested about two days after injury, the closed head injury patients performed below the control group for concrete, but not abstract nouns. Citing previous evidence (cf. Levin et al., 1976a) that short-term memory for complex designs may be disturbed after severe closed head injury, Richardson suggested that damage to the temporal lobes renders patients less capable of utilizing imagery. A plausible competing hypothesis is that mildly injured patients tested shortly after injury have a nonspecific difficulty in attending to features of the words and are thus unable to realize the gain in performance usually afforded by high imagery words.

To summarize, systematic investigation of the effects of memory retraining is a recent development that has yielded mixed findings with no compelling evidence of general effectiveness. Perhaps the most supportive evidence stems from the work of Jones who found facilitation by imagery training in patients with specific impairment of verbal memory, but no enhancement in patients with global amnesic disorder. In view of the heterogeneity in site of localized lesions and severity of diffuse injury which occur in closed head injury, variation in the pattern of residual memory deficit is to be anticipated. It would behoove us then to develop a range of mnemonic techniques and a flexible approach to remediation of memory deficit. In a recent study, the elaboration of mediating stories was found to facilitate memory in predominantly stroke patients (Gianutsos and Gianutsos, 1979). The potential role of neuropharmacologic agents to improve memory warrants study as does the use of electronic devices for periodic cueing of stored information.

Rehabilitation after mild closed head injury

Most published studies of rehabilitation after head injury have focused on severe injuries, particularly those patients falling in the range of severe disability to persistent vegetative state. However, society bears an enormous financial burden because of disability following mild head injury, which is a common condition. In contrast to the general agreement among health professionals favoring rehabilitation after severe closed head injury, opinion is divided concerning not only the mechanism involved in "postconcussional symptoms," but also about strategies for treatment or prevention of the sequelae.

Gronwall (1977) has described a program for monitoring recovery from mild head injury and for the short-term treatment of symptoms. The strategy for assessment and treatment derives from Gronwall's previous studies (described in Chapter 6), demonstrating a transient reduction in capacity for information processing after mild closed head injury. Accordingly, premature resumption of occupational activities, particularly under conditions of time pressure or divided attention, is postulated by Gronwall to result in failure during this period of compromised cognitive efficiency. Irritability, anxiety, and other "postconcussional" symptoms are likely to develop as a consequence of the patient's inability to work at the preinjury level. The degree of dissonance is further increased in cases in which the patient has not been prepared to expect a temporary slowing of cognition or counseled about gradually returning to work.

The results of an initial Paced Auditory Serial Addition Test (PASAT) given soon after clearing of postinjury confusion are used as a guide for vocational counseling. Mildly injured patients who perform on the PASAT at a level within one standard deviation of the normal control group distribution are advised to gradually resume full-time work and are asked to return one month later for a followup examination. Patients evidencing a mild reduction in processing speed on the PASAT are requested to return in one week for a retest before resuming work. Those patients exhibiting impaired capacity for information processing are referred to an outpatient occupational therapy program designed to increase tolerance to fatigue and noise, facilitate working at speed, and increase resistance to distraction. The occupational therapy program introduces increasingly abstract and complex activities that are individually programmed according to the patient's progress. Each patient maintains a personal record of his quantitative scores on the tasks given in the program in order to maximize the amount of feedback. The occupational therapist provides emotional support. Encouragement is also gained from feedback showing progress in the program. Weekly administration of the PASAT provides an index of improvement that is strongly related to resolution of the postconcussional symptoms (Gronwall, 1976b). When the patient's performance approaches the designated criterion score, the next step is to return to part-time work with gradual resumption of a full-time schedule. Gronwall found that practice effects in normal subjects are negligible after the second test and thus progressive improvement may be attributed to physiologic changes.

Of more than 100 closed head injury patients attending the occupational pro-

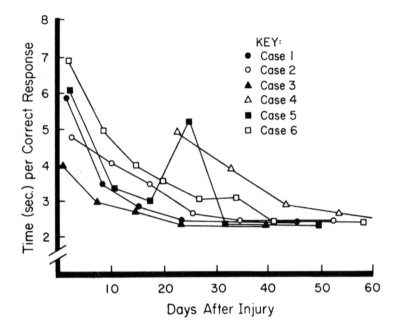

Fig. 11-1. Recovery curves for paced auditory serial addition from six patients who underwent occupational therapy after a mild head injury. [From Gronwall, D.M.A. (1977). Paced auditory serial-addition task: A measure of recovery from concussion. *Percep. Motor Skills* 44:367–373. Reproduced with permission of the author and publisher.]

gram described by Gronwall, 70% returned to work within two weeks of injury. Figure 11-1 shows recovery curves for individuals who attended the rehabilitation program. Deviation from the characteristic pattern of PASAT performance is reported as suggestive of malingering in mildly injured patients. Gronwall's findings indicate that outpatient treatment programs for mild closed head injury deserve further exploration.

12. Some directions for future research

The purpose of this brief concluding chapter is to consider some of the persisting problems that need to be resolved if our understanding of the neuropsychological consequences of traumatic head injury and our effectiveness in treating and rehabilitating the head-injured patient are to be enhanced.

Structural and physiologic changes

One set of problems has to do with the structural and physiologic alterations produced by head injury and how they are related to the behavioral manifestations of the injury. As Chapter 1, on pathophysiologic mechanisms, indicated, the diverse events and phenomena that constitute the neuropathology of head injury (and diffuse microscopic injury of the white matter in particular) are not fully disclosed either by computerized tomography (at least in its present stage of development) or by clinical neurologic indices of structural disease. Given such limitations in defining the extent and severity of a head injury, it is not surprising that correlations between the estimated degree of structural-physiologic alterations and the severity of observed behavioral impairment, although positive and statistically significant, have proven to be relatively modest in degree. It could be concluded that these correlations accurately reflect a true state of affairs, since a patient's behavioral efficiency is determined by diverse factors, including his premorbid personality make-up and his current life situation, as well as by the state of his brain. However, before such a conclusion is accepted, efforts should be made to achieve a more adequate definition of the cerebral alterations associated with head injury.

Direct neurophysiologic approaches, as exemplified by EEG analysis, measurement of cerebral blood flow, and the study of evoked sensory potentials, hold the promise of providing particularly valuable information. The preliminary observations of Obrist and coworkers (1979) on the interrelations of cerebral blood flow, neurologic status, and outcome in head-injured patients and those of Greenberg and coworkers (1977) on the correlations of hemispheric and brain stem sensory potentials with clinical neurologic signs are cases in point. These studies provide a starting point for continuing investigative work that will have to include the collection of reliable normative data to serve as a basis for the interpretation of the findings on head-injured patients. Neurophysiologic findings may prove to be of specific value for elucidating the sometimes puzzling behavioral disturbances following seemingly mild concussion when no evidence of structural damage can be elicited and when, *faute de mieux*, "functional" or motivational determinants are often invoked as an explanation. Among other problems that require attention is that of the relationships between electrophysiologic indices, such as the EEG and evoked potential findings, and the locus and extent of structural pathology, as indicated by CT scan. Nor have the correlations between electroencephalographic findings and the Glasgow Coma Scale ratings been investigated systematically.

Measurement of cerebral metabolism by positron emission tomography (PET) may provide an index of physiologic alteration associated with diffuse and focal effects of closed head injury. This technique offers the possibility of studying the changes in cerebral metabolism that accompany engagement in specific cognitive activities. The PET technique may identify physiologic discontinuities as the patient emerges from coma, as posttraumatic amnesia resolves, and when storage and retrieval of information in long-term memory are recovered. Monitoring changes in specific neurotransmitters during the early phases of recovery from closed head injury could disclose alterations linked to major behavioral disturbances that commonly occur, but that are still poorly understood.

Coma

The first event after a closed head injury is, of course, a period of disturbed consciousness or awareness that may range from momentary confusion to coma of long duration. The measurement of the severity of coma has been advanced significantly by the development of the Glasgow Coma Scale, by Teasdale and Jennett (1974), which has now gained deservedly wide use throughout the world. Yet, problems in the interpretation of the behavior of the comatose patient remain, particularly in respect to the judgment of whether or not a "purposeful" motor response to stimulation has been made and in respect to the global distinction between "consciousness" and "unconsciousness." These problems are very often resolved if successive ratings over a period of 48 to 72 hours are secured. In general, the measurement of change over the first 72 hours seems to provide a more valid index of severity of injury, as well as a sounder basis for prognosis, than does the initial examination on admission to the hospital. In any case, the most effective ways of utilizing the Glasgow Scale and kindred rating schedules deserve exploration.

Outcome

Chapter 3 has summarized the statistics about outcome after closed head injury, both in terms of survival and morbidity. Because of diversity of opinion about what constitutes a "good" recovery, the statistical findings from different studies are hardly comparable. In general, neurosurgeons, who are primarily concerned with the survival of the patient and the prevention of devastating physical and mental impairment, tend to view persisting relatively minor disabilities as of little significance as compared to what might have been the fate of the victim of severe head trauma. On the other hand, rehabilitation specialists are likely to consider these minor disabilities as reflective of a poor outcome if, in fact, they interfere with the patient's interpersonal adjustment and vocational effectiveness.

The four-step Glasgow Outcome Scale of Jennett and Bond (1975) represented an important initial step toward an objective measure of outcome status because it provides stable criteria for judgment. However, there is no doubt that scales of this type are too coarse for the assessment of outcome in individual patients who vary widely in pretraumatic behavioral competence, educational background, and occupation (cf. Levin, Grossman, Rose, and Teasdale, 1979). More detail is required to provide an adequate assessment, both for clinical and research purposes. A variety of currently available rating scales could provide items for the development of a more detailed classification, among them "Activities of Daily Living" (ADL) inventories (Diller, 1979), the Vineland Social Maturity Scale (Doll, 1965), the Adaptive Behavior Scale (Nihara et al., 1974; Lambert et al., 1975), and the Brief Psychiatric Rating Scale of Overall and Gorham (1962).

Posttraumatic and retrograde amnesia

Since its introduction by Russell in 1932, the concept of posttraumatic amnesia, i.e., the interval following injury during which the patient cannot register ongoing events in a memory store, has proved to be a most valuable index of severity of injury and predictor of outcome. Yet, as detailed in Chapter 4, a number of ambiguities surround the concept and these cannot help but limit its usefulness. Measurements of posttraumatic amnesia may or may not include the period of coma. There is the question of whether or not it is important to take into account the "islands of memory" that occur within the period of amnesia. There is the further question of the relative value of retrospective judgment as compared to serial testing during the posttraumatic amnesia period. Finally, the duration of posttraumatic amnesia is often determined by combined measurements of the capacity to retain ongoing events in the strict sense and the accuracy of orientation for time, place, and person, and in fact, Russell (1971) defined the end of the amnesia as the return of normal orientation. However, as Gronwall and Wrightson (1980) have shown, these two aspects of mentation and awareness are not synonymous. Some patients show normal orientation at a time when they are still unable to commit ongoing events to memory and, conversely, some patients remain disoriented after they have gained the capacity to remember events over at least a short period of time. The relative significance of each of these performances in assessment and prediction has still to be determined.

The development of a uniform procedure for assessing posttraumatic amnesia would go far toward enhancing its usefulness as a clinical and research tool and, no doubt, would make more intelligible some of the inconsistent findings reported in the literature. This could be accomplished fairly readily through a consensus of experienced investigators in the field. Although studies have shown that posttraumatic amnesia is a statistically significant predictor of quality of recovery, its prognostic value in the individual, as noted earlier, is still rather limited. The possiblity that the application of a uniform procedure in posttraumatic amnesia assessment, coupled with neurologic findings (e.g., diffuse injury vs. the presence of a mass lesion), will provide a more powerful predictive index should be explored. Finally, as detailed in Chapter 4, the status of specific cognitive functions during posttraumatic amnesia calls for investigation.

The measurement of retrograde amnesia has always been difficult. Assessment is, by definition, retrospective in nature, and inconsistency in report as well as the phenomenon of shrinkage contribute to the unreliability of estimates. These limitations are no doubt responsible in part for the discrepancies in the reports about the relationship of posttraumatic amnesia and retrograde amnesia and the existence of a temporal gradient in the retention of remote personal memories.

Memory functions

Impairment in "memory" is surely the most frequently voiced complaint of the posttraumatic patient and a variety of techniques have been utilized to assess his capacity for learning, retention, recognition, and recall. Curiously, the most widely employed technique, digit span, is a relatively insensitive test, and indeed it is doubtful that the forward repetition of digits should even be considered to be a measure of short-term memory.

Many unresolved problems about memory functions in the patient with closed or penetrating head injury call for investigation. A particularly important one is the relationship between neurologic indices of closed head injury and the severity and specificity of memory impairment. Serial assessment of verbal and visual memory has rarely been reported, particularly in relation to neurologic findings. Whether improved memory function after the period of posttraumatic amnesia reflects a quantitative difference from memory function during posttraumatic amnesia, or whether there is a qualitative change in information processing (e.g., employment of different encoding strategies), has not been determined (cf. Schacter and Crovitz, 1977). The question of how much learning and retention can occur during posttraumatic amnesia remains unanswered. It may be noted that this question has implications for the timing of occupational and physical therapy. For example, evidence of capacity for motor learning during posttraumatic amnesia would suggest that patients could benefit from rehabilitation during this period. The possibility of shifting temporal gradients of retrograde amnesia after head injury remains unexplored.

There is suggestive evidence that memory may be disproportionately impaired in relation to intellectual level and perceptual ability, but no definitive evidence is available. The contribution of related processes, such as capacity for sustained attention, to memory performances is another unexplored area. Further study of the relative impairment of various stages and modalities of memory after closed head injury may prove to be particularly valuable as a basis for the development of useful remedial techniques.

Cognitive functions

The WAIS is the test battery that has been most frequently used in assessing posttraumatic intellectual status and it has provided a basis for comparing the findings of different studies. However, there is considerable question as to whether the WAIS is the most effective instrument for this purpose. Although it does provide a measure of what may be called "general intellectual level," it is not well suited for disclosing specific cognitive defects resulting from focal cerebral dysfunction, such as language deficits, visuoperceptive impairment, or specific memory disorder. As detailed in Chapters 7 and 8, impairment in language and perceptuomotor functions occurs far more frequently after closed head injury than had been assumed.

Disturbances of somesthetic perception in patients with penetrating brain wounds have been the subject of considerable study (cf. Bender et al., 1950; Semmes et al., 1960; Weinstein, 1954). However, virtually no attention has been paid to the status of these functions in patients with closed head injury. Nor have possible alterations in audioperceptual capacities been studied in any detail. Whether the information gained from studies in these areas would have important implications for diagnosis and treatment is an open question, but it would be worthwhile to fill these gaps in knowledge.

Advances in our understanding of the determinants and characteristics of the recovery of cognitive functions in the posttraumatic patient depend, in large part, on posing the appropriate questions. In turn, the possibility of securing adequate answers to these questions depends, in large part, on the availability of relevant assessment techniques. The development and standardization of a test battery specifically designed to provide reliable measures of a number of basic aspects of cognitive function would thus be most useful. Such a battery would surely include tests of short-term recognition memory (cf. Brooks, 1974a,b; Levin, Grossman, and Kelly, 1976a), short-term visual reproductive memory (cf. Benton, 1974), speed of information processing (cf. Gronwall and Sampson, 1974; Gronwall and Wrightson, 1974), visuoperceptive and visuoconstructive abilities (cf. Benton, 1979a; Levin, Grossman, and Kelly, 1977a), and language functions (cf. Heilman, Safran, and Geschwind, 1971; Levin, Grossman, and Kelly, 1976b); an assessment of personality traits (cf. Overall and Gorham, 1962; Overall and Klett, 1972) would also be included.

A cooperative project to develop and standardize such a test battery might well be undertaken. If it were widely adopted, such a battery would be of inestimable value in the assessment of posttraumatic cognitive and personality status, in monitoring the course of recovery, and in evaluating the effects of treatment and rehabilitation. The battery could also be used to determine whether or not the quality of recovery in severely injured patients evacuated and initially treated in a helicopter ambulance differs from that in patients with comparable injuries evacuated by conventional emergency medical services.

The effects of new approaches to controlling raised intracranial pressure (e.g., barbiturate administration) on long-term recovery could be studied. The test findings would also be useful as a guide to the direction that rehabilitation should take. It may be noted in this regard that rehabilitation plans often overlook "subclinical" language impairment, which is not an uncommon sequel of closed head injury (cf. Levin et al., 1981; Sarno, 1980).

Closed head injury in children

It has long been known that the behavioral consequences of head injury differ in adults and children, presumably because of differences in cerebral organization and the greater "plasticity" of the nervous system of the child. Yet, it is evident that no simple generalizations about differences in rate or completeness of recovery are possible. Rather, it appears that the differences in the posttraumatic picture are qualitative as well as quantitative. These qualitative differences should be defined more precisely. The long-term consequences of closed head injury in children have not received the attention that they warrant. There are disturbing indications that many children who are considered to have recovered completely from a head injury in fact suffer from specific cognitive deficits that significantly hamper their academic progress and life adjustment and that, in some cases, behavioral deterioration may occur long after the injury. Thus, the natural history of recovery from head injury in children requires detailed study. After the empirical facts have been established, the determinants of various clinical pictures, as reflected in the developmental status of the nervous system and mechanisms of injury, will need to be investigated.

Rehabilitation

A substantial number of new rehabilitation programs have been established during the past two decades. This development is only a natural, indeed necessary, response to the fact that the rate of survival of patients who have sustained a severe head injury has increased. Although these programs are to be found in every major medical center, they vary widely in size, scope, and effectiveness.

The unsolved problems associated with the rehabilitation of head-injured patients are detailed in Chapter 11. The effectiveness of specific programs, the optimal modes of approach, the development of techniques for alleviating memory deficit, impairment in motor skills, and perceptual defects, and the neurologic correlates of progress are among the problems that call for continued investigation. Computer-assisted memory retrieval and the application of microprocessors to circumvent severe dysarthria warrant closer study. Further investigation is also indicated in the development of effective treatment, whether behavioral or psychopharmacologic, for psychiatric disturbance after head injury. The overall functioning of severely injured patients, and their response to rehabilitation, depends, to a considerable degree, on the appropriateness of their behavior and their appreciation of both residual deficits and functions that are relatively preserved. Critical studies in this field are expensive and time-consuming and sometimes difficult to design. But the steadily growing importance of rehabilitation in the total treatment program for the head-injured patient is sufficient justification for intensive investigation designed to augment its effectiveness.

References

Abernethy, J. (1811). Surgical observation on injuries of the head and on miscellaneous subjects. Vol. 2, Dobson, Philadelphia. [Cited by Gurdjian, E.S. (1973), in *Head Injury from Antiquity to the Present with Special Reference to Penetrating Head Wounds*. Springfield:Charles C. Thomas.]

Adams, F. (1956). *The Extant Works of Aretaeus, the Cappadocian.* London:Sydenham Society.

Adams, J.H., Mitchell, D.E., Graham, D.I., and Doyle, D. (1977). Diffuse brain damage of immediate impact type. *Brain.* 100:489–502.

Akert, K., Orth, O.S., Harlow, H.F., and Schiltz, K.A. (1960). Learned behavior of Rhesus monkeys following neonatal bilateral prefrontal lobotomy. *Science,* 132:1944–1945.

Alajouanine, T. and Lhermitte, F. (1965). Acquired aphasia in children. *Brain,* 88:653–662.

Alajouanine, T., Castaigne, P., Lhermitte, F., Escourolle, R., and Ribaucourt B. de (1957). Étude de 43 cas d'aphasie post-traumatique. *Encéphale;* 46:1–45.

Albert, M.S., Butters, N., and Levin, J. (1979). Temporal gradients in the retrograde amnesia of patients with alcoholic Korsakoff's disease. *Arch. Neurol.,* 36:211–216.

Alliez, J. and Sormani, J. (1967). Reflections on post-traumatic schizophrenia. *Ann. Med.-Psychol.,* 125:1–21.

American Psychiatric Association (1980). *Diagnostic and Statistical Manual of Mental Disorders.* Third Ed. DSM III. Washington, D.C..

Anderson, D.W. and Kalsbeek, W.D. (1980). The National Head and Spinal Cord Injury Survey: Assessment of some uncertainties affecting the findings. *J. Neurosurg.* (Suppl.), 53:32–34.

Anderson, D.W., Kalsbeek, W.D., and Hartwell, T.D. (1980). The National Head and Spinal Cord Injury Survey: Design and methodology. *J. Neurosurg.* (Suppl.), 53:11–18.

Annegers, J.F., Grabow, J.D., Groover, R.V., Laws, E.R., Elveback, L.R., and Kurland, L.T. (1980). Seizures after head trauma: A population study. *Neurology, 30*:683–689.

Annegers, J.F., Grabow, J.D., Kurland, L.T., and Laws, E.R. (1980). The incidence, causes, and secular trends of head trauma in Olmsted County, Minnesota. *Neurology, 30*:912–919.

Arseni, C., Constantinovici, A., Iliescu, D., Dobrotă, I., and Gagea, A. (1970). Considerations on posttraumatic aphasia in peace time. *Psychiatria Neurol. Neurochir.*, 73:105–115.

Artiola i Fortuny, L., Briggs, M., Newcombe, F., Ratcliff, G., and Thomas, C. (1980). Measuring the duration of post traumatic amnesia. *J. Neurol. Neurosurg. Psychiat., 43*:377–379.

Baddeley, A.D. (1976). *The Psychology of Memory.* New York:Basic Books.

Baddeley, A.D. and Warrington, E.K. (1973). Memory coding and amnesia. *Neuropsychologia, 11*:159–165.

Bakay, L. and Glasauer, F.E. (1980). *Head Injury.* Boston:Little, Brown and Company.

Basser, L.S. (1962). Hemiplegia of early onset and the faculty of speech with special reference to the effects of hemispherectomy. *Brain, 85*:427–460.

Bastian, H.C. (1898). *A Treatise on Aphasia and other Speech Defects.* London:H.K. Lewis.

Becker, B. (1975). Intellectual changes after closed head injury. *J. Clin. Psychol., 31*:307–309.

Becker, D.P., Miller, J.D., Ward, J.D., Greenberg, R.P., Young, H.F., and Sakalas, R. (1977). The outcome from severe head injury with early diagnosis and intensive management. *J. Neurosurg., 47*:491–502.

Benayoun, R., Guey, J., and Baurand, C. (1969). Étude corrélative des données cliniques électroencéphalographiques et psychologiques chez des traumatisés cranio-cérébraux. *J. de Psychol. Norm. Pathol., 66*:167–193.

Bender, M.B., Teuber, H.-L., and Battersby, W.S. (1950). Discrimination of weights by men with penetrating lesions of parietal lobes. *Trans. Amer. Neurol. Assoc.* 75:252–255.

Benjamin, R.M. and Thompson, R.F. (1959). Differential effects of cortical lesions in infant and adult cats on roughness discrimination. *Exp. Neurol., 1*:305–321.

Benson, D.F. and Geschwind, N. (1967). Shrinking retrograde amnesia. *J. Neurol. Neurosurg. Psychiat., 30*:539–544.

Benson, D.F., Gardner, H., and Meadows, J.C. (1976). Reduplicative paramnesia. *Neurology, 26*:147–151.

Benton, A.L. (1964). Developmental aphasia and brain damage. *Cortex, 1*:40–52.

Benton, A.L. (1967). Problems of test construction in the field of aphasia. *Cortex, 3*:32–58.

Benton, A.L. (1974). *The Visual Retention Test: Clinical and Experimental Applications.* New York:The Psychological Corporation.

Benton, A.L. (1979a). Visuoperceptive, visuospatial, and visuoconstructive disorders, in

Clinical Neuropsychology. K.M. Heilman and E. Valenstein (eds). New York:Oxford University Press, pp. 186–232.

Benton, A.L. (1979b). Behavioral consequences of closed head injury, in *Central Nervous System Trauma Research Status Report*, G.L. Odom (ed.). NINCDS, National Institutes of Health, Bethesda, pp. 220–231.

Benton, A.L. (1980). The neuropsychology of facial recognition. *Am. Psychol.*, 35:176–186.

Benton, A.L. and Howell, I.L. (1941). The use of psychological tests in the evaluation of intellectual function following head injury: Report of a case of post-traumatic personality disorder. *Psychosom. Med.*, 3:138–151.

Benton, A.L. and Joynt, R.J. (1960). Early descriptions of aphasia. *Arch. Neurol.*, 3:205–221.

Benton, A.L. and Van Allen, M.W. (1968). Impairment of facial recognition in patients with cerebral disease. *Cortex*, 4:344–358.

Benton, A.L., Levin, H.S., and Van Allen, M.W. (1974). Geographic orientation in patients with cerebral disease. *Neuropsychologia*, 12:183–191.

Benton, A.L., Van Allen, M.W., and Fogel, M.L. (1964). Temporal orientation in cerebral disease. *J. Nerv. Ment. Dis.*, 139:110–119.

Black, F.W. (1973). Cognitive and memory performance in subjects with brain damage secondary to penetrating missile wounds and closed head injury. *J. Clin. Psychol.*, 29:441–442.

Black, P., Blumer, D., Wellner, A.M., and Walker, A.E. (1971). The head-injured child: Time-course of recovery, with implications for rehabilitation. *Proceedings of an International Symposium on Head Injuries*, Edinburgh:Churchill Livingstone, pp. 131–137.

Blackburn, H.L. and Benton, A.L. (1955). Simple and choice reaction time in cerebral disease. *Confin. Neurol.*, 15:327–338.

Blau, A. (1936). Mental changes following head trauma in children. *Arch. Neurol. Psychiat.*, 35:723–769.

Blomert, D.M. and Sisler, G.C. (1974). The measurement of retrograde post-traumatic amnesia. *Can. Psychiat. Assoc. J.*, 19:185–192.

Bogen, J.E. (1980). Musical performance during anoxia. *Neurology*, 30:1253.

Boismare, F., Le Poncin, M., and Lefrancois, J. (1977). Mémorisation et catécholamines centrales après un traumatisme cranio- cervical experimental chez le rat: Influence d'une administration d'imipramine. *Psychopharmacology*, 55:251–256.

Bond, M.R. and Brooks, D.N. (1976). Understanding the process of recovery as a basis for the investigation of rehabilitation for the brain injured. *Scand. J. Rehab. Med.*, 8:127–133.

Bowers, S.A. and Marshall, L.F. (1980). Outcome in 200 consecutive cases of severe head injury treated in San Diego County: A prospective analysis. *Neurosurgery*, 6:237–242.

Braakman, R. (1978). Interactions between factors determining prognosis in populations of patients with severe head injury, in *Head Injuries Tumors of the Cerebellar Region*. R.A. Frowein, O. Wilcke, A. Karimi-Nejad, M. Brock, and M. Klinger (eds.). New York:Springer-Verlag, pp. 12–15.

Braakman, R., Gelpke, G.J., Habbema, J.D.F., Maas, A.I.R., and Minderhoud, J.M.

(1980). Systematic selection of prognostic features in patients with severe head injury. *Neurosurgery*, 6:362–370.

Breasted, J.H. (1930). *The Edwin Smith Surgical Papyrus*. Vol. 1. Chicago: University of Chicago Press.

Brenner, C., Friedman, A.P., Merritt, H.H., and Denny-Brown, D.E. (1944). Post-traumatic headache. *J. Neurosurg.*, 1:379–391.

Bricolo, A., Turazzi, S., and Feriotti, F. (1979). Combined clinical and EEG examinations for assessment of severity of acute head injuries. *Acta Neurochir.* (Suppl.), 28:35–39.

Bricolo, A. Turazzi, S., and Feriotti, G. (1980). Prolonged posttraumatic unconsciousness. Therapeutic assets and liabilities. *J. Neurosurg.*, 52:625–634.

Brink, J.D., Garrett, A.L., Hale, W.R., Woo-Sam, J., and Nickel, V.L. (1970). Recovery of motor and intellectual function in children sustaining severe head injuries. *Dev. Med. Child Neurol.*, 12:565–571.

Brink, J.D., Imbus, C., and Woo-Sam, J. (1980). Physical recovery after severe closed head trauma in children and adolescents. *J. Pediat.*, 97:721–727.

Britt, R.H., Herrick, M.K., and Hamilton, R.D. (1977). Traumatic locked-in syndrome. *Ann. Neurol.*, 1:590–592.

Brooks, D.N. (1972). Memory and head injury. *J. Nerv. Ment. Dis.*, 155:350–355.

Brooks, D.N. (1974a). Recognition memory after head injury: A signal detection analysis. *Cortex*, 10:224–230.

Brooks, D.N. (1974b). Recognition memory and head injury. *J. Neurol. Neurosurg. Psychiat.*, 37:794–801.

Brooks, D.N. (1975). Long and short term memory in head injured patients. *Cortex*, 11:329–340.

Brooks, D.N. (1976). Wechsler memory scale performance and its relationship to brain damage after severe closed head injury. *J. Neurol. Neurosurg. Psychiat.*, 39:593–601.

Brooks, D.N. and Baddeley, A.D. (1976). What can amnesic patients learn? *Neuropsychologia*, 14:111–122.

Brooks, D.N., Aughton, M.E., Bond, M.R., Jones, P., and Rizvi, S. (1980). Cognitive sequelae in relationship to early indices of severity of brain damage after severe blunt head injury. *J. Neurol. Neurosurg. Psychiat.*, 43:529–534.

Bruce, D.A. (1978). The pathophysiology of increased intracranial pressure, in *Current Concepts*. Kalamazoo:The Upjohn Company.

Bruce, D.A., Raphaely, R.C., Goldberg, A.I., Zimmerman, R.A., Bilaniuk, L.T., Schut, L., and Kuhl, D.E. (1979). Pathophysiology, treatment and outcome following severe head injury in children. *Child's Brain*, 5:174–191.

Bruce, D.A., Schut, L., Bruno, L.A., Wood, J.H., and Sutton, L.N. (1978). Outcome following severe head injury in children. *J. Neurosurg.*, 48:679–688.

Burger, L.J., Kalvin, N.H., and Smith, J.L. (1970). Acquired lesions of the fourth cranial nerve. *Brain*, 93:567–574.

Buschke, H. and Fuld, P.A. (1974). Evaluating storage, retention, and retrieval in disordered memory and learning. *Neurology*, 24:1019–1025.

Butters, N. and Cermak, L.S. (1980). *Alcoholic Korsakoff's Syndrome. An Information-Processing Approach to Amnesia*. New York:Academic Press.

Cairns, H. (1952). Disturbances of consciousness with lesions of brain-stem and diencephalon. *Brain*, 75:109–146.

Carlsson, C.-A., Von Essen, C., and Löfgren, J. (1968). Factors affecting the clinical course of patients with severe head injuries. Part 1: Influence of biological factors. Part 2: Significance of posttraumatic coma. *J. Neurosurg.*, 29:242–251.

Carroll, J.B., Davies, P., and Richman, B. (1971). *The American Heritage Word Frequency Book*. Boston:Houghton Mifflin.

Cartlidge, N.E.F. (1978). Post-concussional syndrome. *Scott. Med. J.*, 23:103.

Castiglioni, A. (1958). *A History of Medicine*. New York:Alfred A. Knopf.

Caveness, W.F. (1977). Incidence of craniocerebral trauma in the United States, 1970–1975. *Ann. Neurol.*, 1:507.

Caveness, W.F., Meirowsky, A.M., Rish, B.L., Mohr, J.P., Kistler, J.P., Dillon, J.D., and Weiss, G.H. (1979). The nature of posttraumatic epilepsy. *J. Neurosurg.*, 50:545–553.

Cermak, L. and Butters, N. (1972). The role of interference and encoding in the short-term memory deficits of Korsakoff patients. *Neuropsychologia*, 10:89–95.

Chadwick, J. and Mann, W.N. (1950). *The Medical Works of Hippocrates*. Oxford:Blackwell.

Clifton, G.L., Grossman, R.G., Makela, M.E., Miner, M.E., Handel, S., and Sadhu, V. (1980). Neurological course and correlated computerized tomography findings after severe closed head injury. *J. Neurosurg.*, 52:611–624.

Clifton, G.L., Ziegler, M.G., and Grossman, R.G. (1981). Circulating cathecholamines and sympathetic activity after head injury. *Neurosurgery*, 8:10–14.

Corkin, S. (1968). Acquisition of motor skill after bilateral medial temporal-lobe excision. *Neuropsychologia*, 6:225–265.

Corkin, S. (1979). Hidden figures test performance: Lasting effects of unilateral penetrating head injury and transient effect of bilateral cingulotomy. *Neuropsychologia*, 17:585–605.

Cotard, J. (1868). Étude sur l'atrophie cérébrale. Thèse, Paris.

Courville, C.B. (1945). Effects of closed cranial injuries on the midbrain and upper pons, in *Trauma of the Central Nervous System*. Baltimore:Williams & Wilkins, pp. 131–150.

Courville, C.B. (1953). *Commotio Cerebri. Cerebral Concussion and the Postconcussion Syndrome in their Medical and Legal Aspects*. San Francisco:San Lucas.

Craft, A.W. (1972). Head injury in children, in *Handbook of Clinical Neurology*, Vol. 23, P.J. Vinken and G.W. Bruyn (eds.). New York:Elsevier, pp. 445–458.

Craik, F.I.M. and Lockhart, R.S. (1972). Levels of processing: A framework for memory research. *J. Verb. Learn. Verb. Behav.*, 11:671–684.

Craik, F.I.M. and Tulving, E. (1975). Depth of processing and the retention of words in episodic memory. *J. Exp. Psychol.: Gen.*, 104:268–294.

Crompton, M.R. (1970). Visual lesions in closed head injury. *Brain*, 93:785–792.

Crompton, M.R. (1971a). Brainstem lesions due to closed head injury. *Lancet*, 1:669–673.

Crompton, M.R. (1971b). Hypothalamic lesions following closed head injury. *Brain*, 94:165–172.

Cronholm, B. (1972). Evaluation of mental disturbances after head injury. *Scand. J. Rehab. Med.*, 4:35–38.

Cronholm, B. and Jonsson, I. (1957). Memory functions after cerebral concussion. *Acta Chir. Scand.*, 113:263–271.

Crovitz, H.F. (1979). Memory retraining in brain-damaged patients: the airplane list. *Cortex*, 15:131–134.

Crovitz, H.F. and Quina-Holland, K. (1976). Proportion of episodic memories from early childhood by years of age. *Bull. Psychonomic Soc.*, 7:61–62.

Crovitz, H.F. and Schiffman, H. (1974). Frequency of episodic memories as a function of their age. *Bull. Psychonomic Soc.*, 4:517–518.

Crovitz, H.F., Harvey, M.T., and Horn, R.W. (1979). Problems in the acquisition of imagery mnemonics: Three brain-damaged cases. *Cortex*, 15:225–234.

Daniel, P.M. and Treip, C.S. (1966). Lesions of the pituitary gland associated with head injuries, in *The Pituitary Gland*, G.W. Harris and B.T. Donovan (eds.). London:Butterworth, pp. 519–534.

Davidson, P.W., Willoughby, R.H., O'Tuama, L.A., Swisher, C.N., and Benjamins, D. (1978). Neurological and intellectual sequelae of Reye's syndrome. *Am. J. Ment. Defic.*, 82:535–541.

Debray-Ritzen, P., Hirsch, J.-F., Pierre-Kahn, A., Bursztejn, C., and Labbe, J.-P. (1977). Atteinte transitoire du langage écrit en rapport avec un hématome du lobe temporal gauche chez une adolescente de quatorze ans. *Rev. Neurol.*, 133:207–210.

Dee, H.L. and Van Allen, M.W. (1973). Speed of decision-making processes in patients with unilateral cerebral disease. *Arch. Neurol.*, 28:163–166.

Dencker, S.J. (1960). Closed head injury in twins. *Arch. Gen. Psychiat.*, 2:569–575.

Dencker, S.J. and Lofving, B. (1958). A psychometric study of identical twins discordant for closed head injury. *Acta Psychiat. Neurol. Scand.* (Suppl.), 122:119–126.

Denny-Brown, D. (1945). Disability arising from closed head injury. *J.A.M.A.*, 127:429–436.

Denny-Brown, D. and Russell, W.R. (1941). Experimental cerebral concussion, *Brain*, 64:7–164.

Diamond, I.T. and Neff, W.D. (1957). Ablation of temporal cortex and discrimination of auditory patterns. *J. Neurophysiol.*, 20:300–315.

Dikmen, S. and Reitan, R.M. (1976). Psychological deficits and recovery of functions after head injury. *Trans. Am. Neurol. Assoc.*, 101:72–77.

Dikmen, S. and Reitan, R.M. (1977). Emotional sequelae of head injury. *Ann. Neurol.*, 2:492–494.

Dikmen, S. and Reitan, R.M. (1978). Neuropsychological performance in posttraumatic epilepsy. *Epilepsia*, 19:177–183.

Diller, L. (1970). Psychomotor and vocational rehabilitation. In: *Behavioral Changes in Cerebrovascular Disease*. A.L. Benton (ed.), New York:Harper & Row, pp. 81–105.

Dolinskas, C.A., Zimmerman, R.A., Bilaniuk, L.T., and Uzzell, B.P. (1978). Correlation of long-term follow-up neurologic, psychologic, and cranial computed tomographic evaluations of head trauma patients. *Neuroradiology*, 16:318–319.

Doll, E.A. (1965). *Vineland Social Maturity Scale: Manual of Directions*. Minneapolis:Educational Test Bureau.

Drachman, D.A. and Arbit, J. (1966). Memory and the hippocampal complex. *Arch. Neurol.*, 15:52–61.

Dresser, A.C., Meirowsky, A.M., Weiss, G.H., McNeel, M.L., Simon, G.A., and Caveness, W.F. (1973). Gainful employment following head injury. Prognostic factors. *Arch. Neurol.* 29:111–116.

Ebbell, B. (1937). *The Papyrus Ebers*. Copenhagen:Levin and Munksgaard.

Eidelberg, E. and Stein, D.G. (1974). Functional recovery after lesions of the nervous system. *Neurosci. Res. Prog. Bull.*, 12:195–233.

Erickson, R.C. and Scott, M.L. (1977). Clinical memory testing—A review. *Psychol. Bull.*, 84:1130–1141.

Ewing, R., McCarthy, D., Gronwall, D., and Wrightson, P. (1980). Persisting effects of minor head injury observable during hypoxic stress. *J. Clin. Neuropsychol.*, 2:147–155.

Fahy, T.J., Irving, M.H., and Millac, P. (1967). Severe head injuries. *Lancet*, 2:475–479.

Field, J.H. (1976). *Epidemiology of Head Injury in England and Wales:* With particular application to rehabilitation. Leicester:Printed for H.M. Stationery Office by Willsons.

Finger, S. (1978). *Recovery From Brain Damage: Research and Theory*. New York:Plenum Press.

Flach, J. and Malmros, R. (1972). A long-term follow-up study of children with severe head injury. *Scand. J. Rehab. Med.*, 4:9–15.

Fleischer, A.S., Rudman, D.R., Payne, N.S., and Tindall, G.T. (1978). Hypothalamic hypothyroidism and hypogonadism in prolonged traumatic coma. *J. Neurosurg.*, 49:650–657.

Fodor, I.E. (1972). Impairment of memory functions after acute head injury. *J. Neurol. Neurosurg. Psychiat.*, 35:818–824.

Franklin, H.C. and Holding, D.H. (1977). Personal memories at different ages. *Quart. J. Exp. Psychol.*, 29:527–532.

French, B.N. and Dublin, A.B. (1977). The value of computerized tomography in the management of 1000 consecutive head injuries. *Surg. Neurol.*, 7:171–183.

Friedman, A.P., Brenner, C., and Denny-Brown, D. (1945). Post-traumatic vertigo and dizziness. *J. Neurosurg.*, 2:36–46.

Front, D., Beks, J.W.F., Georganas, Ch.L., Beekhuis, H., and Penning, L. (1972). Abnormal patterns of cerebrospinal fluid flow and absorption after head injuries: Diagnosis by isotope cisternography. *Neuroradiology*, 4:6–13.

Fuld, P.A. and Fisher, P. (1977). Recovery of intellectual ability after closed head-injury. *Dev. Med. Child Neurol.*, 19:495–502.

Gaidolfi, E. and Vignolo, L.A. (1980). Closed head injuries of school-age children: Neuropsychological sequelae in early adulthood. *Italian J. Neurol. Sci.*, 1:65–73.

Gama, J.-P. (1835). *Traité des Plaies de Tête et de l'Encéphalite*. Paris:Crochard.

Gardeur, D., Allal, R., Piedelièvre, C., and Metzger, J. (1979). Étude tomodensitométrique des lésions cérébrales post-traumatiques. *J. Radiol.*, 60:79–86.

Gasparrini, B. and Satz, P. (1979). A treatment for memory problems in left hemisphere CVA patients. *J. Clin. Neuropsychol.*, 1:137–150.

Gerstenbrand, F. (1972). The courses of restitution of brain injury in the early and late stages and the rehabilitation measures. *Scand. J. Rehab. Med.*, 4:85–89.

Geschwind, N. (1964). Non-aphasic disorders of speech. *Int. J. Neurol.*, 4:207–214.

Geschwind, N. (1974). *Selected Papers on Language and the Brain*. Dordrecht, Holland:D. Reidel.

Gianutsos, R. and Gianutsos, J. (1979). Rehabilitating the verbal recall of brain-injured patients by mnemonic training: An experimental demonstration using single-case methodology. *J. Clin. Neuropsychol.*, 1:117–135.

Gilchrist, E. and Wilkinson, M. (1979). Some factors determining prognosis in young people with severe head injuries. *Arch. Neurol.*, 36:355–358.

Girard, J. and Marelli, R. (1977). Posttraumatic hypothalamo-pituitary insufficiency. Diagnostic and therapeutic problems in a prepubertal child. *J. Pediat.*, 90:241–242.

Gjone, R., Kristiansen, K., and Sponheim, N. (1972). Rehabilitation in severe head injuries. *Scand. J. Rehab. Med.*, 4:2–4.

Glanzer, M. and Cunitz, A.R. (1966). Two storage mechanisms in free recall. *J. Verb. Learn. Verb. Behav.*, 5:351–360.

Glasgow, R.E., Zeiss, R.A., Barrera, M., Jr., and Lewinsohn, P.M. (1977). Case studies on remediating memory deficits in brain-damaged individuals. *J. Clin. Psychol.*, 33:1049–1054.

Goldman, P.S. (1973). An alternative to developmental plasticity: Heterology of CNS structures in infants and adults, in *Plasticity and Recovery of Function in the Central Nervous System*, D.G. Stein, J.J. Rosen, and N. Butters (eds.). New York:Academic Press, pp. 149–174.

Goldstein, G. (1980). *Rehabilitation of the Brain-Damaged Adult*. New York:Plenum Press.

Goldstein, K. (1942). *Aftereffects of Brain Injuries in War, Their Evaluation and Treatment*. New York:Grune and Stratton.

Goodglass, H. and Kaplan, E. (1972). *The Assessment of Aphasia and Related Disorders*. Philadelphis:Lea and Febiger.

Graham, D.I. and Adams, J.H. (1971). Ischaemic brain damage in fatal head injuries. *Lancet*, 1:265–266.

Granholm, L. and Svendgaard, N. (1972). Hydrocephalus following traumatic head injuries. *Scand. J. Rehab. Med.*, 4:31–34.

Greenberg, R.P., Becker, D.P., Miller, J.D., and Mayer, D.J. (1977). Evaluation of brain function in severe human head trauma with multimodality evoked potentials. Part 2: Localization of brain dysfunction and correlation with posttraumatic neurological conditions. *J. Neurosurg.*, 47:163–177.

Greenberg, R.P., Mayer, D.J., Becker, D.P., and Miller, J.D. (1977). Evaluation of brain function in severe human head trauma with multimodality evoked potentials. Part I: Evoked brain-injury potentials, methods, and analysis. *J. Neurosurg.*, 47:150–162.

Griffith, D. and Actkinson, T.R. (1978). Mental aptitude and mnemonic enhancement. *Bull. Psychonomic Soc.*, 12:347–348.

Groher, M. (1977). Language and memory disorders following closed head trauma. *J. Speech Hear. Res.*, 20:212–223.

Gronwall, D. (1976a). Concussion: Does intelligence help? *NZ Psychologist*, 5:72–78.

Gronwall, D. (1976b). Performance changes during recovery from closed head injury. *Proc. Austral. Assoc. Neurol.*, 13:143–147.

Gronwall, D. (1977). Paced auditory serial-addition task: A measure of recovery from concussion. *Percept. Mot. Skills*, 44:367–373.

Gronwall, D. and Sampson, H. (1974). *The Psychological Effects of Concussion*. Auckland:Auckland University Press.

Gronwall, D. and Wrightson, P. (1974). Delayed recovery of intellectual function after minor head injury. *Lancet*, 2:605–609.

Gronwall, D. and Wrightson, P. (1975). Cumulative effect of concussion. *Lancet*, 2:995–997.

Gronwall, D. and Wrightson, P. (1980). Duration of post-traumatic amnesia after mild head injury. *J. Clin. Neuropsychol.* 2:51–60.

Groslambert, R., Perret, J., and Boucharlat, J. (1965). Confusion mentale posttraumatique lors d'une contusion du lobe temporal droit. *J. Med. Lyon*, 46:641–643.

Grossman, R.G. (1979) Electrophysiologic evaluation of the central nervous system after trauma, in *Central Nervous System Trauma Research Status Report*, G.L. Odom (ed.). NINCDS, National Institute of Health, Bethesda: pp. 155–177.

Grossman, R., Beyer, C., Kelly, P., and Haber, B. (1975). Acetylcholine and related enzymes in human ventricular and subarachnoid fluids following brain injury. *Proceedings of the Fifth Annual Meeting of the Society for Neuroscience*, 76.3:506.

Grossman, R.G., Lindquist, C., Feinstein, R., and Eisenberg, H.M. (1979). Monitoring of the excitability of the cerebral cortex in brain injury with the direct cortical response, in *Neural Trauma*, A.J. Popp (ed.). New York:Raven Press, pp. 237–243.

Groswasser, Z., Mendelson, L., Stern, M.J., Schechter, I., and Najenson, T. (1977). Reevaluation of prognostic factors in rehabilitation after severe head injury. Assessment thirty months after trauma. *Scand. J. Rehab. Med.*, 9:147–149.

Gruszkiewicz, J., Doron, Y., and Peyser, E. (1973). Recovery from severe craniocerebral injury with brain stem lesions in childhood. *Surg. Neurol.*, 1:197–201.

Gurdjian, E.S. (1971). Mechanisms of impact injury of the head, in *Head Injuries. Proceedings of an International Symposium held in Edinburgh and Madrid*. Edinburgh:Churchill Livingstone, pp. 17–22.

Gurdjian, E.S. (1973). *Head Injury From Antiquity to the Present with Special Reference to Penetrating Head Wounds*. Springfield:Charles C. Thomas.

Gurdjian, E.S. and Gurdjian, E.S. (1976). Cerebral contusions: Reevaluation of the mechanism of their development. *J. Trauma*, 16:35–51.

Gurdjian, E.S. and Webster, J.E. (1958). *Head Injuries: Mechanisms, Diagnosis, and Management*. Boston:Little, Brown and Company.

Guttman, E. (1942). Aphasia in children. *Brain*, 65:205–219.

Guttman, E. (1946). Late effects of closed head injuries: Psychiatric observations. *J. Ment. Sci.*, 92:1–18.

Guyotat, J., Dumas, R., and Marie-Cardine, M. (1968). Psychiatric hospitalization after cranial trauma. *J. Med. Lyon, 49*:629–649.

Hadley, E.E. (1922). The mental symptom complex following cranial trauma. *J. Nerv. Ment. Dis., 56*:567–590.

Hall, G.W. (1925). The relation of psychotic and neurotic disturbances to head injuries. *Illinois Med. J., 48*:279–286.

Hamsher, K., Levin, H.S., and Benton, A.L. (1979). Facial recognition in patients with focal brain lesions. *Arch. Neurol., 36*:837–839.

Hannay, H.J., Levin, H.S., and Grossman, R.G. (1979). Impaired recognition memory after head injury. *Cortex, 15*:269–283.

Hannay, H.J., Levin, H.S., and Kay, M. (1981). Tachistoscopic visual perception after closed head injury. *J. Clin. Neuropsychol.*, In press.

Hawthorne, V.M. (1978). Epidemiology of head injuries. *Scott. Med. J., 23*:92.

Hécaen, H. (1976). Acquired aphasia in children and the ontogenesis of hemispheric functional specialization. *Brain and Language, 3*:114–134.

Heilman, K.M., Safran, A., and Geschwind, N. (1971). Closed head trauma and aphasia. *J. Neurol. Neurosurg. Psychiat., 34*:265–269.

Heiskanen, O. and Kaste, M. (1974), Late prognosis of severe brain injury in children. *Dev. Med. Child Neurol., 16*:11–14.

Hendrick, E.B., Harwood-Hash, D.C.F., and Hudson, A.R. (1964). Head injuries in children: A survey of 4465 consecutive cases at the Hospital for Sick Children, Toronto, Canada. *Clin. Neurosurg., 11*:46–59.

Higashi, K., Sakata, Y., Hatano, M., Abiko, S., Ihara, K., Katayama, S., Wakuta, Y., Okamura, T., Ueda, H., Zenke, M., and Aoki, H. (1977). Epidemiological studies on patients with a persistent vegetative state. *J. Neurol. Neurosurg. Psychiat., 40*:876–885.

Hillbom, E. (1951). Schizophrenia-like psychoses after brain trauma. *Acta Psychiatr. Scand.* (Suppl.), *60*:36–47.

Hjern, B. and Nylander, I. (1964). Late prognosis of severe head injuries in childhood. *Acta Paediatr. Scand.* (Suppl.), *152*:113–116.

Holbourn, A.H.S. (1943). Mechanics of head injuries. *Lancet, 2*:438–441.

Höök, O. (1976). Rehabilitation, in *Handbook of Clinical Neurology*, Vol. 24, P.J. Vinken and G.W. Bruyn (eds.). Amsterdam:North-Holland Publishing Co., pp. 683–697.

Jamison, D.L. and Kaye, H.H. (1974). Accidental head injury in children. *Arch. Dis. Childhood, 49*:376–381.

Jennett, B. (1972). Head injuries in children. *Dev. Med. Child Neurol., 14*:137–147.

Jennett, B. (1975). Who cares for head injuries? *Br. Med. J., 3*: 267–270.

Jennett, B. (1976a). Resource allocation for the severely brain damaged. *Arch. Neurol., 33*:595–597.

Jennett, B. (1976b). Assessment of the severity of head injury. *J. Neurol. Neurosurg. Psychiat., 39*:647–655.

Jennett, B. (1979). Posttraumatic epilepsy. *Adv. Neurol., 22*:137–147.

Jennett, B. and Bond, M. (1975). Assessment of outcome after severe brain damage. *Lancet, 1*:480–487.

Jennett, B. and Plum, F. (1972). Persistent vegetative state after brain damage. *Lancet,* 1:734–737.

Jennett, B. and Teasdale, G. (1981). *Management of Head Injuries.* Philadelphia:F.A. Davis Company.

Jennett, B., Teasdale, G., Braakman, R., Minderhoud, J., Heiden, J., and Kurze, T. (1979). Prognosis of patients with severe head injury. *Neurosurgery,* 4:283–289.

Jennett, B., Teasdale, G., Braakman, R., Minderhoud, J., and Knill- Jones, R. (1976). Predicting outcome in individual patients after severe head injury. *Lancet,* 1:1031–1034.

Jennett, B., Teasdale, G., Galbraith, S., Pickard, J., Grant, H., Braakman, R., Avezaat, C., Maas, A., Minderhoud, J., Vecht, C.J., Heiden, J., Small, R., Caton, W., and Kurze, T. (1977). Severe head injuries in three countries. *J. Neurol. Neurosurg. Psychiat.,* 40:291–298.

Jennett, B., Teasdale, G., and Knill-Jones, R. (1975). Prognosis after severe head injury, in *CIBA Outcome of Severe Damage to the CNS.* New York:Elsevier, pp. 309–320.

Jennett, W.B. (1969). Head injuries and the temporal lobe, in *Current Problems in Neuropsychiatry,* R.N. Herrington (ed.). *Br. J. Psychiat.,* special publication No 4. Ashford, Kent, United Kingdom: Headley Brothers Ltd.

Johnson, D. and Almli, C.R. (1978). Age, brain damage, and performance, in *Recovery from Brain Damage: Research and Theory,* S. Finger, (ed.). New York:Plenum Press, pp. 115–132.

Jones, M.K. (1974). Imagery as a mnemonic aid after left temporal lobectomy: Contrast between material-specific and generalized memory disorders. *Neuropsychologia,* 12:21–30.

Kalsbeek, W.D., McLaurin, R.L., Harris, B.S.H., III, and Miller, J.D. (1980). The National Head and Spinal Cord Injury Survey: Major Findings. *J. Neurosurg.* (Suppl.), 53:19–31.

Kennard, M.A. (1938). Reorganization of motor functions in the cerebral cortex of monkeys deprived of motor and premotor areas in infancy. *J. Neurophysiol.,* 1:477–497.

Kerr, T.A., Kay, D.W.K., and Lassman, L.P. (1971). Characteristics of patients, type of accident, and mortality in a consecutive series of head injuries admitted to a neurosurgical unit. *Br. J. Prev. Soc. Med.,* 25:179–185.

Kimura, D. (1963). Right temporal-lobe damage. *Arch. Neurol.,* 8:264–271.

Kishore, P.R.S., Lipper, M.H., Miller, J.D., Girevendulis, A.K., Becker, D.P., and Vines, F.S. (1978). Posttraumatic hydrocephalus in patients with severe head injury. *Neuroradiology,* 16:261–265.

Klonoff, H. (1971). Head injuries in children: Predisposing factors, accident conditions, accident proneness and sequelae. *Am. J. Public Health,* 61:2405–2417.

Klonoff, H. and Low, M. (1974). Disordered brain function in young children and early adolescents: Neuropsychological and electroencephalographic correlates, in *Clinical Neuropsychology: Current Status and Applications,* R.M. Reitan and L.A. Davison (eds.). New York:John Wiley and Sons.

Klonoff, H. and Paris, R. (1974). Immediate, short-term and residual effects of acute head injuries in children: neuropsychological and neurological correlates, in *Clinical Neuropsychology: Current Status and Applications*, R.M. Reitan and L.A. Davison (eds.). New York:John Wiley and Sons, pp. 179–210.

Klonoff, H. and Thompson, G.B. (1969). Epidemiology of head injuries in adults: A pilot study. *Canad. Med. Assoc. J.*, 100:235–241.

Klonoff, H., Low, M.D., and Clark, C. (1977). Head injuries in children: A prospective five year follow-up. *J. Neurol. Neurosurg. Psychiat.*, 40:1211–1219.

Kløve, H. and Cleeland, C.S. (1972). The relationship of neuropsychological impairment to other indices of severity of head injury. *Scand. J. Rehab. Med.*, 4:55–60.

Kobrine, A.I., Timmins, E., Rajjoub, R.K., Rizzoli, H.V., and Davis, D.O. (1977). Demonstration of massive traumatic brain swelling within 20 minutes after injury. Case Report. *J. Neurosurg.*, 46:256–258.

Kornblum, R.N. and Fisher, R.S. (1969). Pituitary lesions in craniocerebral injuries. *Arch. Path.*, 88:242–248.

Kraus, J.F. (1980a). A comparison of recent studies on the extent of the head and spinal cord injury problem in the United States. *J. Neurosurg.* (Suppl.), 53:35–43.

Kraus, J.F. (1980b). Injury to the head and spinal cord: The epidemiological relevance of the medical literature published from 1960 to 1978. *J. Neurosurg.* (Suppl.), 53:3–10.

Kreindler, A., Arseni, C., and Mihailescu, L. (1975). Aphasia following non-missile injury of the brain. *Rev. Roum. Med.-Neurol. Psychiat.*, 13:247–254.

Kremer, M., Russell, W.R., and Smyth, G.E. (1947) A mid-brain syndrome following head injury. *J. Neurol. Neurosurg. Psychiat.*, 10:49–60.

Lambert, N.M., Windmiller, M., Cole, L., and Figueroa, R. (1975). *AAMD Adaptive Behavior Scale—Public School Version*. Washington, D.C.:American Association for Mental Deficiency.

Landau, W.M., Goldstein, R., and Kleffner, F.R. (1960). Congenital aphasia: A clinicopathologic study. *Neurology*, 10:915–921.

Lange-Cosack, H. and Tepfer, G. (1973). *Das Hirntrauma im Kindes und Jugendalter*. New York:Springer.

Lange-Cosack, H., Wider, B., Schlesner, H.-J., Grumme, Th., and Kubicki, St. (1979). Prognosis of brain injuries in young children (one until five years of age). *Neuropaediatrie*, 10:105–127.

Langfitt, T.W. (1978). Measuring the outcome from head injuries. *J. Neurosurg.*, 48:673–678.

Langfitt, T. (1981). A holistic view of head injury including a new classification, in *Neural Trauma*, Fourth Symposium, R.G. Grossman and P.L. Gildenberg (eds.). New York:Raven Press (in press).

Lanksch, W., Grumme, T., and Kazner, E. (1979). *Computed Tomography in Head Injuries*. New York:Springer-Verlag.

Levin, H.S. and Benton, A.L. (1975). Temporal orientation in patients with brain disease. *Appl. Neurophysiol.*, 38:56–60.

Levin, H.S. and Eisenberg, H.M. (1979a). Neuropsychological outcome of closed head injury in children and adolescents. *Child's Brain*, 5:281–292.

Levin, H.S. and Eisenberg, H.M. (1979b). Neuropsychological impairment after closed head injury in children and adolescents. *J. Pediatr. Psychol.*, 4:389–402.

Levin, H.S. and Eisenberg, H.M. (1979c). Verbal learning and memory in relation to focal and diffuse effects of closed head injury. Paper presented at Academy of Aphasia Meeting, 16 October 1979, San Diego, California.

Levin, H.S. and Grossman, R.G. (1976). Effects of closed head injury on storage and retrieval in memory and learning of adolescents. *J. Pediatr. Psychol.*, 1:38–42.

Levin, H.S. and Grossman, R.G. (1978). Behavioral sequelae of closed head injury: A quantitative study. *Arch. Neurol.*, 35:720–727.

Levin, H.S. and Peters, B.H. (1976). Neuropsychological testing following head injuries: Prosopagnosia without visual field defect. *Dis. Nerv. Syst.*, 37:68–71.

Levin, H.S., Grossman, R.G., and Kelly, P.J. (1976a). Short-term recognition memory in relation to severity of head injury. *Cortex*, 12:175–182.

Levin, H.S., Grossman, R.G., and Kelly, P.J. (1976b). Aphasic disorder in patients with closed head injury. *J. Neurol. Neurosurg. Psychiat.*, 39:1062–1070.

Levin, H.S., Grossman, R.G., and Kelly, P.J. (1977a). Impairment of facial recognition after closed head injuries of varying severity. *Cortex*, 13:119–130.

Levin, H.S., Grossman, R.G., and Kelly, P.J. (1977b). Assessment of long-term memory in brain damaged patients. *J. Consult. Clin. Psychol.*, 45:684–688.

Levin, H.S., Grossman, R.G., Rose, J.E., and Teasdale, G. (1979). Long-term neuropsychological outcome of closed head injury. *J. Neurosurg.*, 50:412–422.

Levin, H.S., Grossman, R.G., Sarwar, M., and Meyers, C.A. (1981). Linguistic recovery after closed head injury. *Brain and Language*, 12:360–374.

Levin, H.S., Hamsher, K., and Benton, A.L. (1975). A short form of the test of facial recognition for clinical use. *J. Psychol.*, 91:223–228.

Levin, H.S., Meyers, C.A., Grossman, R.G., and Sarwar, M. (1981). Ventricular enlargement after closed head injury. *Arch. Neurol.*, 38:623–629.

Levin, H.S., O'Donnell, V.M., and Grossman, R.G. (1979). The Galveston orientation and amnesia test: A practical scale to assess cognition after head injury. *J. Nerv. Ment. Dis.*, 167:675–684.

Levin, H.S., Peters, B.H., and Hulkonen, D.A. (1982). Early concepts of anterograde and retrograde amnesia. *Cortex* (in press).

Lewin, W. (1968). Rehabilitation after head injury. *Br. Med. J.*, 1:465–470.

Lewinsohn, P.M., Danaher, B.G., and Kikel, S. (1977). Visual imagery as a mnemonic aid for brain-injured persons. *J. Consult. Clin. Psychol.*, 45:717–723.

Lewis, A.J. (1976). *Mechanisms of Neurological Disease*. Boston:Little, Brown and Company.

Lezak, M.D. (1976). *Neuropsychological Assessment*. New York:Oxford University Press.

Lezak, M.D. (1979). Recovery of memory and learning functions following traumatic brain injury. *Cortex*, 15:63–72.

Lhermitte, J., Massary, J. de, and Huguenin, R. (1929). Syndrome occipital avec alexie pure d'origine traumatique, par. *Rev. Neurol.*, 2:703–707.

Lindenberg, R. and Freytag, E. (1970). Brainstem lesions characteristic of traumatic hyperextension of the head. *Arch. Path.*, 90:509–515.

Lindenberg, R., Fisher, R.S., Durlacher, S.H., Lovitt, W.V., Jr., and Freytag, E. (1955).

Lesions of the corpus callosum following blunt mechanical trauma to the head. *Am. J. Path., 31*:297–317.

Lishman, W.A. (1973). The psychiatric sequelae of head injury: A review. *Psychol. Med., 3*:304–318.

Lockhart, R.S. and Murdock, B.B., Jr. (1970). Memory and the theory of signal detection. *Psychol. Bull., 74*:100–109.

London, P.S. (1967). Some observations on the course of events after severe injury of the head. *Ann. Roy. Coll. Surg. Engl., 41*:460–479.

Lundholm, J., Jepsen, B.N., and Thornval, G. (1975). The late neurological, psychological, and social aspects of severe traumatic coma. *Scand. J. Rehab. Med., 7*:97–100.

Luria, A.R. (1968). *The Mind of a Mnemonist.* New York:Basic Books, Inc.

Maccoby, E.M. and Jacklin, C.N. (1974). *The Psychology of Sex Differences.* Stanford:Stanford University Press.

Major, R.H. (1954). *A History of Medicine.* Vols. I and II. Springfield:Charles C. Thomas.

Maki, Y., Akimoto, H., and Enomoto, T. (1980). Injuries of basal ganglia following head trauma in children. *Child's Brain, 7*:113–123.

Mandleberg, I.A. (1975). Cognitive recovery after severe head injury. 2. Wechsler Adult Intelligence Scale during post-traumatic amnesia. *J. Neurol. Neurosurg. Psychiat., 38*:1127–1132.

Mandleberg, I.A. (1976). Cognitive recovery after severe head injury. 3. WAIS verbal and performance IQ's as a function of post-traumatic amnesia duration and time from injury. *J. Neurol. Neurosurg. Psychiat., 39*:1001–1007.

Mandleberg, I.A. and Brooks, D.N. (1975). Cognitive recovery after severe head injury. I. Serial testing on the Wechsler Adult Intelligence Scale. *J. Neurol. Neurosurg. Psychiat., 38*:1121–1126.

Marshall, L.F., Smith, R.W., and Shapiro, H.M. (1979a). The outcome with aggressive treatment in severe head injuries. Part 1: The significance of intracranial pressure monitoring. *J. Neurosurg., 50*:20–25.

Marshall, L.F., Smith, R.W., and Shapiro, H.M. (1979b). The outcome with aggressive treatment in severe head injuries. Part II: Acute and chronic barbiturate administration in the management of head injury. *J. Neurosurg., 50*:26–30.

Marslen-Wilson, W.D. and Teuber, H.-L. (1975). Memory for remote events in anterograde amnesia: Recognition of public figures from news-photographs. *Neuropsychologia, 13*:353–364.

Martin, G. (1974). *A Manual of Head Injuries in General Surgery.* London:William Heinemann Medical Books, Ltd.

Maury, M., Audic, B., Lacombe, M., and Lucet, G. (1970). La rééducation des traumatisés craniens. *Ann. Méd. Physique, 13*:47–59.

Meadows, J.C. (1974). The anatomical basis of prosopagnosia. *J. Neurol. Neurosurg. Psychiat., 37*:489–501.

Merskey, H. and Woodforde, J.M. (1972). Psychiatric sequelae of minor head injury. *Brain, 95*:521–528.

Mesulam, M.-M., Waxman, S.G., Geschwind, N., and Sabin, T.D. (1976). Acute confusional states with right middle cerebral artery infarctions. *J. Neurol. Neurosurg. Psychiat.*, 39:84–89.

Mettler, C.C. (1947). *History of Medicine; A Correlative Text, Arranged According to Subjects*, F.A. Mettler (ed.). Philadelphia:Blakiston.

Meyer, A. (1904). The anatomical facts and clinical varieties of traumatic insanity. *Am. J. Insanity*, 60:373–441.

Miller, E. (1970). Simple and choice reaction time following severe head injury. *Cortex*, 6:121–127.

Miller, E. (1980). The training characteristics of severely head- injured patients: A preliminary study. *J. Neurol. Neurosurg. Psychiat.*, 43:525–528.

Miller, H. (1961). Accident neurosis. *Br. Med. J.*, 1:919–925, 992–998.

Miller, J.D., Becker, D.P., Ward, J.D., Sullivan, H.G., Adams, W.E., and Rosner, M.J. (1977). Significance of intracranial hypertension in severe head injury. *J. Neurosurg.*, 47:503–516.

Miller, J.D., Butterworth, J.F., Gudeman, S.K., Faulkner, J.E., Choi, S.C., Selhorst, J.B., Harbison, J.W., Lutz, H.A., Young, H.F., and Becker, D.P. (1981). Further experience in the management of severe head injury. *J. Neurosurg.*, 54:289–299.

Miller, J.D., Sweet, R.C., Narayan, R., and Becker, D.P. (1978). Early insults to the injured brain. *J.A.M.A.*, 240:439–442.

Milner, B. (1974). Sparing of language functions after early unilateral brain damage. *Neurosci. Res. Prog. Bull.*, 12:213–217.

Milner, B. (1978). Clues to the cerebral organization of memory, in *Cerebral Correlates of Conscious Experience INSERM Symposium No. 6*, P.A. Buser and A. Rougeul-Buser (eds.). New York:ElsevierNorth-Holland Biomedical Press, pp. 139–153.

Mitchell, D.E. and Adams, J.H. (1973). Primary focal impact damage to the brainstem in blunt head injuries. Does it exist? *Lancet*, 2:215–218.

Moore, B.E. and Ruesch, J. (1944). Prolonged disturbances of consciousness following head injury. *N. Engl. J. Med.*, 230:445–452.

Morsier, G. de (1973). Sur 23 cas d'aphasie traumatique. *Psychiat. Clin.*, 6:226–239.

Najenson, T., Groswasser, Z., Stern, M., Schechter, I., Daviv, C., Berghaus, N., and Mendelson, L. (1975). Prognostic factors in rehabilitation after severe head injury. *Scand. J. Rehab. Med.*, 7:101–105.

Najenson, T., Mendelson, L., Schechter, I., Daviv, C., Mintz, N., and Groswasser, Z. (1974). Rehabilitation after severe head injury. *Scand. J. Rehab. Med.*, 6:5–14.

Najenson, T., Sazbon, L., Fiselzon, J., Becker, E., and Schechter, I. (1978). Recovery of communicative functions after prolonged traumatic coma. *Scand. J. Rehab. Med.*, 10:15–21.

Natelson, B.H., Haupt, E.J., Fleischer, E.J., and Grey, L. (1979). Temporal orientation and education. A direct relationship in normal people. *Arch. Neurol.*, 36:444–446.

Natelson, S.E. and Sayers, M.P. (1973). The fate of children sustaining severe head trauma during birth. *Pediatrics*, 51:169–174.

Naughton, J.A.L. (1971). The effects of severe head injuries in children. Psychological aspects. *Proceedings of an International Symposium on Head Injuries*. Edinburgh:Churchill Livingstone, pp. 106–110.

Newcombe, F. (1969). *Missile Wounds of the Brain: A Study of Psychological Deficits*. New York:Oxford University Press.

Nihara, K., Foster, R., Shellhaas, M., and Leland, H. (1974). *AAMD Adaptive Behavior Scale*. Washington, D.C.:American Association for Mental Deficiency.

Norrman, B. and Svahn, K. (1961). A follow-up study of severe brain injuries. *Acta Psychiat. Scand.*, 37:236–264.

Obrist, W.D., Gennarelli, T.A., Segawa, H., Dolinskas, C.A., and Langfitt, T.W. (1979). Relation of cerebral blood flow to neurological status and outcome in head-injured patients. *J. Neurosurg.*, 51:292–300.

Oddy, M. and Humphrey, M. (1980). Social recovery during the year following severe head injury. *J. Neurol. Neurosurg. Psychiat.*, 43:798–802.

Oddy, M., Humphrey, M., and Uttley, D. (1978). Subjective impairment and social recovery after closed head injury. *J. Neurol. Neurosurg. Psychiat.*, 41:611–616.

Oka, H., Kako, M., Matsushima, M., and Ando, K. (1977). Traumatic spreading depression syndrome. Review of a particular type of head injury in 37 patients. *Brain*, 100:287–298.

Ommaya, A.K. and Gennarelli, T.A. (1974). Cerebral concussion and traumatic unconsciousness: Correlation of experimental and clinical observations on blunt head injuries. *Brain*, 97:633–654.

Oppenheimer, D.R. (1968). Microscopic lesions in the brain following head injury. *J. Neurol. Neurosurg. Psychiat.*, 31:299–306.

Orbach, J. and Fantz, R.L. (1958). Differential effects of temporal neo-cortical resections on overtrained and non-overtrained visual habits in monkeys. *J. Comp. Physiol. Psychol.*, 51:126–129.

Overall, J.E. and Gorham, D.R. (1962). The brief psychiatric rating scale. *Psychol. Repos.*, 10:799–812.

Overall, J.E. and Klett, C.J. (1972). *Applied Multivariate Analysis*. New York:McGraw-Hill.

Paivio, A. (1971). *Imagery and Verbal Processes*. New York:Holt, Rinehart and Winston.

Patten, B.M. (1972). The ancient art of memory. Usefulness in treatment. *Arch. Neurol.*, 26:25–31.

Paxson, C.L. and Brown, D.R. (1976). Post-traumatic anterior hypopituitarism. *Pediatrics*, 57:893–896.

Peacher, W.G. (1945). Speech disorders in World War II. II. Further studies. *J. Nerv. Ment. Dis.*, 102:165–171.

Peters, B.H. and Levin, H.S. (1977). Memory enhancement after physostigmine treatment in the amnesic syndrome. *Arch. Neurol.*, 34:215–219.

Peterson, L.R. and Peterson, M.J. (1959). Short-term retention of individual verbal items. *J. Exp. Psychol.*, 58:193–198.

Plum, F. and Posner, J. (1980). *The Diagnosis of Stupor and Coma*. Philadelphia:F.A. Davis Company.

Povlishock, J.T., Becker, D.P., Kontos, H.A., and Jenkins, L.W. (1979). Neural and vascular alterations in brain injury, in *Neural Trauma*, A.J. Popp, R.S. Bourke, L.R. Nelson, and H.K. Kimelbert (eds.). New York:Raven Press, pp. 79–93.

Pudenz, R.H. and Shelden, C.H. (1946). The lucite calvarium—A method for direct observation of the brain; II. Cranial trauma and brain movement. *J. Neurosurg.*, 3:487–505.

Rappaport, M., Hopkins, K., Hall, K., Belleza, T., and Berrol, S. (1978). Brain evoked potential use in a physical medicine and rehabilitation setting. *Scand. J. Rehab. Med.*, 10:27–32.

Rappaport, M., Hall, K., Hopkins, K., Belleza, T., Berrol, S., and Reynolds, G. (1977). Evoked brain potentials and disability in brain-damaged patients. *Arch. Phys. Med. Rehab.*, 58:333–338.

Renfrew, E.L. (1971). An approach to the severe head injury. *Physiotherapy*, 57:50–60.

Reyes, R.L., Bhattacharyya, A.K., and Heller, D. (1981). Traumatic head injury: Restlessness and agitation as prognosticators of physical and psychologic improvement in patients. *Arch. Phys. Med. Rehab.*, 62:20–23.

Ribot, T. (1882). *Diseases of Memory: An Essay in the Positive Psychology*. New York:Appleton.

Richardson, F. (1963). Some effects of severe head injury. A follow-up study of children and adolescents after protracted coma. *Dev. Med. Child Neurol.*, 5:471–482.

Richardson, J.T. (1979a). Mental imagery, human memory, and the effects of closed head injury. *Br. J. Soc. Clin. Psychol.*, 18:319–327.

Richardson, J.T. (1979b). Signal detection theory and the effects of severe head injury upon recognition memory. *Cortex*, 15:145–148.

Roberts, A.H. (1980). *Severe Accidental Head Injuries. An Assessment of Long-Term Prognosis*. Baltimore:University Park Press.

Robertson, R.C.L. and Pollard, C., Jr. (1955). Decerebrate state in children and adolescents. *J. Neurosurg.*, 12:13–17.

Robinson, J.A. (1976). Sampling autobiographical memory. *Cognitive Psychol.*, 8:578–595.

Rockoff, M.A., Marshall, L.F., and Shapiro, H.M. (1979). High-dose barbiturate therapy in humans: A clinical review of 60 patients. *Ann. Neurol.*, 6:194–199.

Romano, M.D. (1974). Family response to traumatic head injury. *Scand. J. Rehab. Med.*, 6:1–4.

Rosenbaum, M., Lipsitz, N., Abraham, J., and Najenson, T. (1978). A description of an intensive treatment project for the rehabilitation of severely brain-injured soldiers. *Scand. J. Rehab. Med.*, 10:1–6.

Rosin, A.J. (1977). Reactions of families of brain-injured patients who remain in a vegetative state. *Scand. J. Rehab. Med.*, 9:1–5.

Rosin, A.J. (1978). Very prolonged unresponsive state following brain injury. *Scand. J. Rehab. Med.*, 10:33–38.

Rowbotham, G.F., Maciver, I.N., Dickson, J., and Bousfield, M.E. (1954). Analysis of 1,400 cases of acute injury to the head. *Br. Med. J.*, 1:726–730.

Rubens, A.B., Geschwind, N., Mahowald, M.W., and Mastri, A. (1977). Posttraumatic cerebral hemispheric disconnection syndrome. *Arch. Neurol.*, 34:750–755.

Ruesch, J. (1944a). Dark adaptation, negative after images, tachistoscopic examinations and reaction time in head injuries. *J. Neurosurg.*, 1:243–251.

Ruesch, J. (1944b). Intellectual impairment in head injuries. *Am. J. Psychiat.*, 100:480–496.

Ruesch, J. and Bowman, K.M. (1945). Prolonged post-traumatic syndromes following head injury. *Am. J. Psychiat.*, *102*:145–163.

Ruesch, J. and Moore, B.E. (1943). Measurement of intellectual functions in the acute stage of head injury. *Arch. Neurol.*, *50*:165–170.

Rune, V. (1970). Acute head injuries in children. A retrospective, epidemiologic, and electroencephalographic study on primary school children in Umea. *Acta Paediatr. Scand.*, *209*:3–12.

Rusk, H.A., Block, J.M., and Lowman, E.W. (1969). Rehabilitation of the brain-injured patient: A report of 157 cases with long-term follow-up of 118, in *The Late Effects of Head Injury*, A.E. Walker, W.F. Caveness, and M. Critchley (eds.). Springfield:Charles C. Thomas, pp. 327–332.

Rusk, H.A., Lowman, E.W., and Block, J.M. (1966). Rehabilitation of the patient with head injuries. *Clin. Neurosurg.*, *12*:312–323.

Russell, W.R. (1932). Cerebral involvement in head injury. *Brain*, *55*:549–603.

Russell, W.R. (1935). Amnesia following head injuries. *Lancet*, *2*:762–763.

Russell, W.R. (1947). The neurology of brain wounds. *Br. J. Surg.*, *War Surg.* (Suppl.), *1*:250–252.

Russell, W.R. (1960). Injury to cranial nerves and optic chiasm, in *Injuries of the Brain and Spinal Cord and Their Coverings*, 4th Ed., S. Brock (ed.). New York:Springer-Verlag, pp. 118–126.

Russell, W.R. (1971). *The Traumatic Amnesias*. New York:Oxford University Press.

Russell, W.R. and Espir, M.L.E. (1961). *Traumatic Aphasia. A Study of Aphasia in War Wounds of the Brain*. New York:Oxford University Press.

Russell, W.R. and Nathan, P.W. (1946). Traumatic amnesia. *Brain*, *69*:183–187.

Russell, W.R. and Smith, A. (1961). Post-traumatic amnesia in closed head injury. *Arch. Neurol.*, *5*:4–17.

Rutherford, W.H., Merrett, J.D., and McDonald, J.R. (1977). Sequelae of concussion caused by minor head injuries. *Lancet*, *1*:1–4.

Sanders, H.I. and Warrington, E.K. (1971). Memory for remote events in amnesic patients. *Brain*, *94*:661–668.

Sarno, M.T. (1980). The nature of verbal impairment after closed head injury. *J. Nerv. Ment. Dis.*, *168*:685–692.

Savino, P.J., Glaser, J.S., and Schatz, N.J. (1980). Traumatic chiasmal syndrome. *Neurology*, *30*:963–970.

Schacter, D.L. and Crovitz, H.F. (1977). Memory function after closed head injury: A review of the quantitative research. *Cortex*, *13*:150–176.

Scharlock, D.P., Neff, W.D., and Strominger, N.L. (1965). Discrimination of tone duration after bilateral ablation of cortical auditory areas. *J. Neurophysiol.*, *28*:673–681.

Scharlock, D.P., Tucker, T.J., and Strominger, N.L. (1963). Auditory discrimination by the cat after neonatal ablation of temporal cortex. *Science*, *141*:1197–1198.

Schilder, P. (1934). Psychic disturbances after head injuries. *Am. J. Psychiat.*, *91*:155–188.

Schnaper, N. and Cowley, R.A. (1976). Overview: Psychiatric sequelae to multiple trauma. *Am. J. Psychiat.*, *133*:883–890.

Schott, B., Michel, F., Michel, D., and Dumas, R. (1969). Apraxie idéomotrice unilatérale gauche avec main gauche anomique: Syndrome de déconnexion calleuse? *Rev. Neurol.*, *120*:359–365.

Scoville, W.B. and Milner, B. (1957). Loss of recent memory after bilateral hippocampal lesions. *J. Neurol. Neurosurg. Psychiat.*, *20*:11–21.

Seales, D.M., Rossiter, V.S., and Weinstein, M.E. (1979). Brainstem auditory evoked responses in patients comatose as a result of blunt head trauma. *J. Trauma*, *19*:347–353.

Selecki, B.R., Hoy, R.J., and Ness, P. (1967). A retrospective survey of neuro-traumatic admissions to a teaching hospital: Part 1. General aspects. *Med. J. Aust.*, *2*:113–117.

Selecki, B.R., Hoy, R.J., and Ness, P. (1968). Neurotraumatic admissions to a teaching hospital: A retrospective survey. Part 2. Head injuries. *Med. J. Aust.*, *1*:851–855.

Seltzer, B. and Benson, D.F. (1974). The temporal pattern of retrograde amnesia in Korsakoff's disease. *Neurology*, *24*:527–530.

Semmes, J., Weinstein, S., Ghent, L., and Teuber, H.-L. (1960). *Somatosensory Changes after Penetrating Brain Wounds in Man.* Cambridge:Harvard University Press.

Shaffer, D., Chadwick, O., and Rutter, M. (1975). Psychiatric outcome of localized head injury in children, in *Outcome of Severe Damage to the Central Nervous System*, Ciba Foundation Symposium 34 (new series). Amsterdam:Elsevier, Excerpta Medica, North-Holland.

Shapiro, L.B. (1939). Schizophrenic-like psychosis following head injuries. *Ill. Med. J.*, *76*:250–254.

Sisler, G. and Penner, H. (1975). Amnesia following severe head injury. *Can Psychiat. Assoc. J.*, *20*:333–336.

Smith, A. and Sugar, O. (1975). Development of above normal language and intelligence 21 years after left hemispherectomy. *Neurology*, *25*:813–818.

Smith, E. (1974). Influence of site of impact on cognitive impairment persisting long after severe closed head injury. *J. Neurol. Neurosurg. Psychiat.*, *37*:719–726.

Snoek, J., Jennett, B., Adams, J.H., Graham, D.I., and Doyle, D. (1979). Computerised tomography after recent severe head injury in patients without acute intracranial haematoma. *J. Neurol. Neurosurg. Psychiat.*, *42*:215–225.

Spreen, O. and Benton, A.L. (1969). *Neurosensory Center Comprehensive Examination for Aphasia: Manual of Directions.* Victoria, B.C.:Neuropsychology Laboratory, University of Victoria.

Squire, L.R. (1974). Remote memory as affected by aging. *Neuropsychologia*, *12*:429–435.

Squire, L.R. and Slater, P.C. (1975). Forgetting in very long-term memory as assessed by an improved questionnaire technique. *J. Exp. Psychol: Human Learning and Memory*, *1*:50–54.

Squire, L.R. and Slater, P.C. (1978). Anterograde and retrograde memory impairment in chronic amnesia. *Neuropsychologia*, *16*:313–322.

Starr, A. (1978). Sensory evoked potentials in clinical disorders of the nervous system. *Ann. Rev. Neurosci.*, *1*:103–127.

Steadman, J.H. and Graham, J.G. (1970). Rehabilitation of the brain- injured. *Proc. R. Soc. Med.*, 63:23–28.

Stengel, E. (1947). A clinical and psychological study of echo-reactions. *J. Ment. Sci.*, 93:598–612.

Stern, J.M. (1978). Cranio-cerebral injured patients. *Scand. J. Rehab. Med.*, 10:7–10.

Steudel, W.I. and Krüger, J. (1979). Using the spectral analysis of the EEG for prognosis of severe brain injuries in the first post-traumatic week. *Acta Neurochir.* (Suppl.), 28:40–42.

Stone, J.L., Lopes, J.R., and Moody, R.A. (1978). Fluent aphasia after closed head injury. *Surg. Neurol.*, 9:27–29.

Stover, S.L. and Zeiger, H.E., Jr. (1976). Head injury in children and teenagers: Functional recovery correlated with the duration of coma. *Arch. Physical Med. Rehab.*, 57:201–205.

Strauss, I. and Savitsky, N. (1934). Head injury. *Arch. Neurol.*, 31:893–895.

Strich, S.J. (1956). Diffuse degeneration of the cerebral white matter in severe dementia following head injury. *J. Neurol. Neurosurg. Psychiat.*, 19:163–185.

Strich, S.J. (1969). The pathology of brain damage due to blunt head injuries, in *The Late Effects of Head Injury*, A.E. Walker, W.F. Caveness, and M. Critchley (eds.). Springfield:Charles C. Thomas, pp. 501–526.

Strich, S.J. (1970). Lesions in the cerebral hemispheres after blunt head injury, in *The Pathology of Trauma*, S. Sevitt and H.B. Stoner (eds.). London:BMA House, pp. 166–171.

Sweet, R.C., Miller, J.D., Lipper, M., Kishore, P.R.S., and Becker, D.P. (1978). Significance of bilateral abnormalities on the CT scan in patients with severe head injury. *Neurosurgery*, 3:16–21.

Symonds, C. (1966). Disorders of memory. *Brain*, 89:625–644.

Symonds, C. (1962). Concussion and its sequelae. *Lancet*, 1:1–5.

Takahashi, H. and Nakazawa, S. (1980). Specific type of head injury in children. Report of 5 cases. *Child's Brain*, 7:124–131.

Taylor, A.R. and Bell, T.K. (1966). Slowing of cerebral circulation after concussional head injury. *Lancet*, 2:178–180.

Teasdale, G. (1976). Assessment of head injuries. *Br. J. Anaesth.*, 48:761–766.

Teasdale, G. and Jennett, B. (1974). Assessment of coma and impaired consciousness: A practical scale. *Lancet*, 2:81–84.

Teasdale, G. and Jennett, B. (1976). Assessment and prognosis of coma after head injury. *Acta Neurochir.*, 34:45–55.

Teasdale, G., Knill-Jones, R., and Van Der Sande, J. (1978). Observer variability in assessing impaired consciousness and coma. *J. Neurol. Neurosurg. Psychiat.*, 41:603–610.

Teuber, H.-L. (1969). Neglected aspects of the posttraumatic syndrome, in *The Late Effects of Head Injury*, A.E. Walker, W.F. Caveness, and M. Critchley (eds.). Springfield:Charles C. Thomas, pp. 13–34.

Teuber, H.-L. (1975). Recovery of function after brain injury in man, in *Outcome of Severe Damage to the Central Nervous System*, Ciba Foundation Symposium 34 (new series). Amsterdam:Elsevier, Excerpta Medica, North-Holland, pp. 159–190.

Teuber, H.-L. (1978). The brain and human behavior, in *Perception*, R. Held, H.W. Leibowitz, and H.-L. Teuber (eds.). New York:Springer-Verlag, pp. 879–920.

Thomsen, I.V. (1974). The patient with severe head injury and his family. *Scand. J. Rehab. Med.*, 6:180–183.

Thomsen, I.V. (1975). Evaluation and outcome of aphasia in patients with severe closed head trauma. *J. Neurol. Neurosurg. Psychiat.*, 38:713–718.

Thomsen, I.V. (1976). Evaluation and outcome of traumatic aphasia in patients with severe verified focal lesions. *Folia Phoniat.*, 28:362–377.

Thomsen, I.V. (1977). Verbal learning in aphasic and non-aphasic patients with severe head injuries. *Scand. J. Rehab. Med.*, 9:73–77.

Thomsen, I.V. and Skinhoj, E. (1976). Regressive language in severe head injury. *Acta Neurol. Scandinav.*, 54:219–226.

Todorow, S. (1975). Recovery of children after severe head injury. Psychoreactive superimpositions. *Scand. J. Rehab. Med.*, 7:93–96.

Todorow, S. and Heiss, E. (1978). The "fall asleep syndrome", a kind of secondary disturbance of consciousness after head injury, in *Head Injuries: Tumors of the Cerebellar Region*, R.A. Frowein, O. Karimi-Nejad, M. Brock, and M. Klinger (eds.). New York:Springer-Verlag, pp. 102–104.

Toglia, J.U. (1972). Vestibular and medico-legal aspects of closed cranio-cervical trauma. *Scand. J. Rehab. Med.*, 4:126–132.

Tucker, T.J., Kling, A., and Scharlock, D.P. (1968). Sparing of photic frequency and brightness discriminations after striatectomy in neonatal cats. *J. Neurophysiol.*, 31:818–832.

Tulving, E. and Colotla, V.A. (1970). Free recall of trilingual lists. *Cognitive Psychol.*, 1:86–98.

Uzzell, B.P., Zimmerman, R.A., Dolinskas, C.A., and Obrist, W.D. (1979). Lateralized psychological impairment associated with CT lesions in head injured patients. *Cortex*, 15:391–401.

Van Dongen, K.J. and Braakman, R. (1980). Late computed tomography in survivors of severe head injury. *Neurosurgery*, 7:14–22.

Van Woerkom, T.C.A.M., Teelken, A.W., and Minderhoud, J.M. (1977). Difference in neurotransmitter metabolism in frontotemporal-lobe contusion and diffuse cerebral contusion. *Lancet*, 1:812–813.

Van Zomeren, A.H. and Deelman, B.G. (1978). Long-term recovery of visual reaction time after closed head injury. *J. Neurol. Neurosurg. Psychiat.*, 41:452–457.

Vapalahti, M. and Troupp, H. (1971). Prognosis for patients with severe brain injuries. *Br. Med. J.*, 3:404–407.

Vigouroux, R.P. (1971). Les traumatismes cranio-faciaux. *Neurochirurgie*, 17:245–290.

Vigouroux, R.P., Baurand, C., Choux, M., and Guillermain, P. (1972). État actual des aspects séquellaires graves dans les traumatismes craniens de l'adulte. *Neurochirurgie* (Suppl. 2), 18:1–260.

Von Wowern, F. (1966). Posttraumatic amnesia and confusion as an index of severity in head injury. *Acta Neurol. Scand.*, 42:373–378.

Warrington, E.K. and James, M. (1967). An experimental investigation of facial recognition in patients with unilateral cerebral lesions. *Cortex*, 3:317–326.

Warrington, E.K. and Sanders H.I. (1971). The fate of old memories. *Quart. J. Exp. Psychol.*, *23*:432–442.

Warrington, E.K. and Weiskrantz, L. (1968). A study of learning and retention in amnesic patients. *Neuropsychologia*, *6*:238–291.

Warrington, E.K. and Weiskrantz, L. (1970). Amnesic syndrome: Consolidation or retrieval? *Nature*, *228*:628–630.

Watkins, M.J. (1974). Concept and measurement of primary memory. *Psychol. Bull.*, *81*:695–711.

Wechsler, D. and Stone, C.P. (1945). *Wechsler Memory Scale*. New York:Psychological Corp.

Weingartner, H. (1978). Human state dependent learning, in *Drug Discrimination and State Dependent Learning*, B.T. Ho, D.W. Richards, III, and D.L. Chute (eds.). New York:Academic Press, pp. 361–382.

Weingartner, H., Miller, H., and Murphy, D.L. (1977). Mood-state-dependent retrieval of verbal associations. *J. Abnorm. Psychol.*, *86*:276–288.

Weinstein, E.A. and Kahn, R.L. (1955). *Denial of Illness; Symbolic and Physiological Aspects*. Springfield:Charles C. Thomas.

Weinstein, E.A. and Keller, N.J.A. (1963). Linguistic patterns of misnaming in brain injury. *Neuropsychologia*, *1*:79–90.

Weinstein, E.A. and Lyerly, O.G. (1968). Confabulation following brain injury. *Arch. Gen. Psychiat.*, *18*:348–354.

Weinstein, S. (1954). Weight judgment in somesthesis after penetrating injury to the brain. *J. Comp. Physiol. Psychol.* *48*:203–207.

Weinstein, S. and Teuber, H.-L. (1957). Effects of penetrating brain injury on intelligence test scores. *Science*, *125*:1036–1037.

Whitely, A.M. and Warrington, E.K. (1977). Prosopagnosia: A clinical, psychological, and anatomical study of three patients. *J. Neurol. Neurosurg. Psychiat.*, *40*:395–403.

WHO (1978). *The International Classification of Diseases: Clinical Modification. ICD-9-CM*. 9th Revn. Vol. 1, Diseases: Tabular List. Ann Arbor:Edwards Brothers, Inc.

Wickelgreen, W.A. (1975). Dynamics of retrieval, in *Short-Term Memory*, D. Deutsch and J.A. Deutsch (eds.). New York:Academic Press, pp. 235–253.

Wilson, P.J.E. (1970). Cerebral hemispherectomy for infantile hemiplegia. A report of 50 cases. *Brain*, *93*:147–180.

Winick, M. (1976). *Malnutrition and Brain Development*. New York:Oxford University Press.

Woods, B.T. and Carey, S. (1979). Language deficits after apparent clinical recovery from childhood aphasia. *Ann. Neurol.*, *6*:405–409.

Yarnell, P.R. and Lynch, S. (1970). Progressive retrograde amnesia in concussed football players: Observation shortly postimpact. *Neurology*, *20*:416.

Yates, F.A. (1966). *The Art of Memory*. Chicago:University of Chicago Press.

Zimmerman, R.A. and Bilaniuk, L.T. (1979). Computed tomography in diffuse traumatic cerebral injury, in *Neural Trauma*, A.J. Popp, R.S. Bourke, L.R. Nelson, and H.K. Kimelbert (eds.). New York:Raven Press, pp. 253–262.

Zimmerman, R.A., Bilaniuk, L.T., Bruce, D., Dolinskas, C., Obrist, W., and Kuhl, D. (1978). Computed tomography of pediatric head trauma: Acute general cerebral swelling. *Radiology*, *126*:403–408.

Zimmerman, R.A., Bilaniuk, L.T., Dolinskas, C., Genneralli, T., Bruce, D., and Uzzel, B. (1977). Computed tomography of acute intracerebral hemorrhagic contusion. *Comput. Axial Tomog.*, *1*:271–280.

Appendix A. Followup interview

Name _____ Age _____ Sex _____

Date of birth _____ Date of injury _____ Education _____

Address _____ UH# _____

_____ Phone _____

Date of test _____ Assessment (months) _____

1. Presently employed   _____
   (1) yes (2) no (3) N.K.

2. Type of work _____

   _____

   (1) same as preinjury (2) less demanding (3) sheltered
   (4) unemployed (5) homemaker (9) N.K.   _____

3. Part or full time (1) full (2) part (3) unemployed
   (9) N.K.   _____

4. Income (1) patient (2) spouse (3) children   Primary   _____
   (4) extended family (5) private insurance   Secondary _____
   (6) WCI (7) unemployment (8) public assist.   Tertiary   _____
   (9) investments (10) SSI (11) court award   Fourth   _____
   (99) N.K.

5. Employment history
                          Position   Dates/Time   Part/Full

Prior to injury			
Prior to injury			
Prior to injury			
Since injury			
Since injury			
Current			

6. Disability/Compensation: Type _____ Amount _____
   (1) Yes   (2) No   (3) N.K.

7. Managing Household Chores   (1) No decline
      (2) Improvement
      (3) Mild decline
      (4) Mod/marked decline
      (5) N.K.   _____

8. Legal dispute   (1) No
      (2) Patient initiated
      (3) Against patient
      (4) 2 and 3
      (5) N.K.   _____

9. Transportation   (1) Alone
      (2) Accompanied
      (3) None
      (4) N.K.   _____

10. Arrests (other than minor traffic violations)
    (1) No   (2) Yes   (9) N.K.   _____

11. Complete if answer to #10 is yes
    Preinjury: juvenile arrest/conviction/crime   _____/_____/_____
            adult   arrest/conviction/crime   _____/_____/_____
    Postinjury: juvenile arrest/conviction/crime   _____/_____/_____
            adult   arrest/conviction/crime   _____/_____/_____
    Arrest: (1) none   (2) one arrest   (3) more than one arrest
    Crime: (1) none   (2) violent with victim
            (3) nonviolent with victim   (4) victimless
            (5) 1 and 2   (6) 1 and 3   (7) 2 and 3   (8) 1, 2, and 3

Compare to Preinjury   *Compare to Last Visit*

12. Dizziness   _____   _____
    (1) No change
    (2) Mild increase
    (3) Mod/marked increase
    (4) Decrease
    (9) N.K.

13. Coordination   _____   _____
    (1) No change
    (2) Mild decrease
    (3) Mod/marked decrease
    (4) Improvement
    (9) N.K.

Compare to Preinjury   *Compare to Last Visit*

14. Headaches   _____   _____
    (1) None
    (2) No increase
    (3) Increase not interfering with daily activities
    (4) Increase interfering with daily activities
    (9) N.K.

15. Vision   _____   _____
    (1) No change
    (2) Mild disturbance
    (3) Mod/marked disturbance
    (4) Improvement
    (9) N.K.

16. Hearing   _____   _____
    (1) No change
    (2) Mild disturbance
    (3) Mod/marked disturbance
    (4) Improvement
    (9) N.K.

17. Taste and Smell   _____   _____
    (1) No change
    (2) Mild decrease
    (3) Mod/marked decrease
    (4) Improvement
    (9) N.K.

18. Seizures   _____   _____
    (1) None
    (2) Preinjury disorder
    (3) At time of impact/acute hospitalization
    (4) After initial hospitalization
    (5) 3 and 4
    (9) N.K.

19. Thinking (efficiency)   _____   _____
    (1) No decline
    (2) Mild decline
    (3) Mod/marked decline
    (4) Improvement
    (9) N.K.

20. Concentration   _____   _____
    (1) No decline
    (2) Mild decline
    (3) Mod/marked decline
    (4) Improvement
    (9) N.K.

Compare to preinjury   *Compare to last visit*

21. Recent memory
    (1) No decline
    (2) Mild decline
    (3) Mod/marked decline
    (4) Improvement
    (9) N.K.

22. Remote memory
    (1) No decline
    (2) Mild decline
    (3) Mod/marked decline
    (4) Improvement
    (9) N.K.

23. Depression
    (1) None
    (2) Mild
    (3) Mod/marked
    (4) Improved
    (9) N.K.

24. Appetite
    (1) No change
    (2) Increased
    (3) Decreased
    (9) N.K.

25. Sleeping
    (1) No change
    (2) Increased
    (3) Sleep disturbance
    (9) N.K.

26. Energy level
    (1) No change
    (2) Increased
    (3) Decreased
    (9) N.K.

27. Sexual Functioning
    (1) No change
    (2) Mild decrease activity/arousal
    (3) Mod/marked decrease
    (4) Increase
    (9) N.K.

Compare to preinjury   *Compare to last visit*

28. Anxiety   _____   _____
    (1) No change
    (2) Mild increase
    (3) Mod/marked increase
    (4) Decrease
    (9) N.K.

29. Patience   _____   _____
    (1) No change
    (2) Mild decrease
    (3) Mod/marked decrease
    (4) Increase
    (9) N.K.

30. Temper/Impulse control   _____   _____
    (1) No change
    (2) Worse
    (3) Better
    (9) N.K.

31. Hallucinations   _____   _____
    (1) None
    (2) Auditory
    (3) Visual
    (4) Auditory and visual
    (9) N.K.

32. Preinjury psychiatric   _____   _____
    (1) None
    (2) Yes, did not seek help
    (3) Outpatient treatment
    (4) Hospitalization
    (9) N.K.

33. Postinjury psychiatric   _____   _____
    (1) None
    (2) Yes, did not seek help
    (3) Outpatient treatment
    (4) Hospitalization
    (9) N.K.

34. Preinjury marital status _____   Present marital status _____
    (1) Single
    (2) Married/cohabiting
    (3) Separated
    (4) Divorced
    (5) Widowed

Compare to preinjury   *Compare to last visit*

35. Duration of marital status (years) _____/_____

36. How getting along with spouse?   _____   _____
    (1) As well as before
    (2) Better than before
    (3) Not as well
    (4) Does not apply

37. How getting along with
    family/friends?   _____   _____
    (1) As well as before
    (2) Better than before
    (3) Not as well
    (4) Does not apply

38. Social activities   _____   _____
    (1) As much as before
    (2) More than before
    (3) Less than before
    (4) Hardly at all

39. Sports/Recreation   _____   _____
    (1) As much as before
    (2) More than before
    (3) Less than before
    (4) Hardly at all

40. Improvement since
    hospitalization   Since last visit
    Physical   _____   _____
    Mental   _____   _____
    (1) Improved
    (2) No change
    (3) Declined
    (9) N.K.

41. Back to normal physically   _____
                   mentally   _____
    (1) Yes
    (2) No
    (3) Unsure
    (9) N.K.

                                    Preinjury   *Postinjury*

42. Drug Use   _____   _____
    Marijuana   _____   _____
    Hallucinogens   _____   _____

	Preinjury	*Postinjury*
Stimulants (Cocaine, amphetamines)	_____	_____
Sedatives/hypnotics (Qualudes, barbiturates)	_____	_____
Narcotics	_____	_____
Minor tranquilizers	_____	_____
Prescription	_____	_____
Other	_____	_____

(1) No   (2) Yes

45. Alcohol Use   _____   _____
    (1) None
    (2) Occasional
    (3) Moderate (less than 2 drinks per day)
    (4) Heavy (more than 2 drinks per day)
    (5) Drinking interfering with job/social functioning

46. Patient reliable   _____   _____
    (1) Yes   (2) No   (3) N.K.

47. Glasgow Recovery Scale   _____   _____
    (1) Good Recovery
    (2) Moderate disability
    (3) Severe disability
    (4) Persistent vegetative state
    (5) N.K.

Appendix B. Galveston Orientation and Amnesia Test (GOAT)

Name _____

Age _____ Sex M F

Date of Birth _____
mo day yr

Diagnosis _____

Date of Test _____
mo day yr

Day of the week s m t w th f s

Time _____ AM PM

Date of injury _____
mo day, yr

GALVESTON ORIENTATION & AMNESIA TEST (GOAT)

Error Points

1. What is your name? (2) _____ When were you born? (4) _____

   Where do you live? (4) _____ ⏋

2. Where are you now? (5) city _____ (5) hospital _____ ⏋

   (unnecessary to state name of hospital)

3. On what date were you admitted to this hospital? (5) _____

   How did you get here? (5) _____ ⏋

4. What is the first event you can remember _after_ the injury? (5) _____

   Can you describe in detail (e.g., date, time, companions) the first event you can recall after injury? (5) _____ ⏋

5. Can you describe the last event you recall _before_ the accident? (5) _____

   Can you describe in detail (e.g., date, time, companions) _____

   the first event you can recall _before_ the injury? (5) _____ ⏋

6. What time is it now? _____ (−1 for each ½ hour removed from correct time to maximum of −5) ⏋

7. What day of the week is it? _____ (−1 for each day removed from correct one) ⏋

8. What day of the month is it? _____ (−1 for each day removed from correct date to maximum of −5) ⏋

9. What is the month? _____ (−5 for each month removed from correct one to maximum of −15) ⏋

10. What is the year? _____ (−10 for each year removed from correct one to maximum of −30) ⏋

Total Error Points ⏋

Total Goat Score (100-total error points)

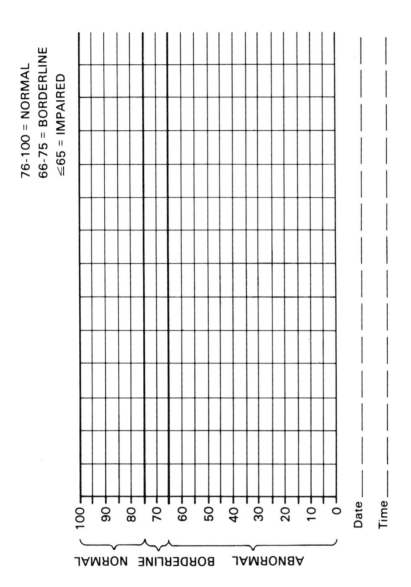

76-100 = NORMAL
66-75 = BORDERLINE
≤65 = IMPAIRED

100 90 80 70 60 50 40 30 20 10 0

Date _____ _____ _____
Time _____ _____ _____

NORMAL BORDERLINE ABNORMAL

Instructions for Scoring the GOAT

Questions

1. Assign 2 error points if patient fails to state first and last names correctly; 4 points if patient fails to state date of birth correctly; 4 points are scored if patient fails to state the town of his residence (street address is unnecessary). A maximum of 10 error points could be scored and entered in the two columns on the extreme right side of the test form.
2. If the patient is unable to state the town he is in at the time of the assessment, 5 points are scored; 5 additional points are deducted if the patient fails to state that he is in the hospital, although mentioning the name of the hospital is unnecessary.
3. Five error points are given if the patient is unable to recall the date of admission; 5 additional points are deducted if the patient fails to describe accurately the mode of transporation to the hospital.
4. Five error points are given when the patient is unable to recall the first event after injury (e.g., waking up in hospital room); patients who cannot recall an event after the injury would have 5 additional error points deducted because of failure to present details of such an event. Those patients who describe a verifiable or at least plausible post-traumatic event, but are unable to provide details, would accrue 5 error points on this question.
5. Criteria for scoring responses are similar to those used in question 4; 5 error points are deducted for vague recall of an event prior to the injury (e.g., driving a car shortly before the accident), whereas 5 additional points are deducted for total failure to recall any retrograde event.
6. Score 1 error point for each half hour that the patient's response deviates from the correct time, up to a maximum of -5.
7. Assign 1 error point for each day that the patient's response is removed from the correct day of the week.
8. Score 1 error point for each day of the month that the patient's response deviates from the correct date, to a maximum of -5.
9. Five error points are deducted for each month that the patient's response is removed from the correct month, to a maximum of -15.
10. Ten error points are deducted for each year that the patient's response deviates from the correct one, to a maximum of -30.

Computation of GOAT Score

Enter the total error points accrued for the 10 items in the lower right hand corner of the test form. The GOAT score equals 100 minus total error points.

Name Index

Subject Index

Acceleration
 deceleration and, 8
 linear, 8
 rotational, 8
 shear strains and, 10
 temporal lobes and, 14
Acute stage of closed head injury
 assessment of injury in, 33–44
 neurologic deficit, 33–40
Age. *See also* Epidemiology of closed head
  injury
 brain plasticity and, 190–92
 of head-injured patients, 55
 orbitofrontal lesions following injury and,
  191
 relationship to incidence of head injury, 55
 relationship to postconcussional syndrome,
  206
 relationship to recovery from head injury,
  64, 66
Agitation. *See* Psychiatric consequences of
  head injury; Recovery from head injury,
  subacute phase
Alcohol. *See* Epidemiology of closed head
  injury; Outcome of head injury;
  Psychiatric consequences of head injury
Amnesia, posttraumatic (anterograde), 73–79
 behavioral manifestations of, 79, 173–76
 cognitive recovery and, 87–89, 137–39
 coma and, 74, 76–77
 confabulation and, 79, 175

definition of, 73–75
 disorientation and, 77–78
 duration of, 73–75, 78–79, 86–87
 hematoma and, 75
 as an index of severity of injury, 73, 78–79
 learning during, 90–91
 measurement of, 75, 91–98
 memory during, 89–90
 outcome of injury, and, 78, 86–87
 prognostic significance of, 74–75, 78, 86–
  87, 175
 reduplicative paramnesia and, 79
 retrograde amnesia and, 73–75, 79–80
 temporal lobe injury and, 73
Amnesia, retrograde, 79–84
 autobiographical memory, 84–85
 correspondence to posttraumatic amnesia,
  79–80
 measurement of, 82–85
 shrinking, 81–82
 temporal gradient in, 82–85
Anatomic changes following head injury,
  223–24
Anosmia, 30
Anterograde amnesia. *See* Amnesia,
  posttraumatic
Aphasia. *See also* Speech and speech
  disturbance
 akinetic mutism and, 151
 anomic, 143, 147–49
 base rate of, 140–41

271